*Living Safe*

- A "Situational Awareness" exercise from Certified Emergency Manager Randall C. Duncan
- A complete blueprint for preparing your Family Disaster Plan
- The most up-to-date information on bears, snake bites, and other subjects for which advice given a few years ago no longer applies
- Both natural and technological disasters
- Fun facts and sobering statistics
- Information that's so current, it's taken from today's headlines. . . .

"The American Red Cross believes that everyone should be prepared for any possible disruption in their daily lives that may be caused by disasters, from a home fire to something that affects the entire community. The content of this book can help you and your family be more prepared and safer should disaster strike. Most steps recommended in this book are simple and easy to do, with little time and effort, yet will result in greater peace of mind for everyone in the family."

—Rocky Lopes, Ph.D.
Sr. Associate for Disaster Education
American Red Cross Headquarters

# LIVING SAFE
## IN AN
# UNSAFE WORLD

*The Complete Guide to
Family Preparedness*

## KATE KELLY

*With an Introduction by
Randall C. Duncan,
Certified Emergency Manager*

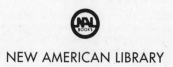

NEW AMERICAN LIBRARY

NAL Books
Published by New American Library, a division of
Penguin Putnam Inc., 375 Hudson Street, New York, New York 10014, U.S.A.
Penguin Books Ltd, 27 Wrights Lane, London W8 5TZ, England
Penguin Books Australia Ltd, Ringwood, Victoria, Australia
Penguin Books Canada Ltd, 10 Alcorn Avenue, Toronto, Ontario, Canada M4V 3B2
Penguin Books (N.Z.) Ltd, 182–190 Wairau Road, Auckland 10, New Zealand

Penguin Books Ltd, Registered Offices: Harmondsworth, Middlesex, England

First published by New American Library,
a division of Penguin Putnam Inc.

First Printing, August 2000
1   3   5   7   9   10   8   6   4   2

(NAL) REGISTERED TRADEMARK—MARCA REGISTRADA

New American is a trademark of Penguin Putnam Inc.

Printed in the United States of America

Set in Cheltenham Light
Designed by Eve L. Kirch

LIBRARY OF CONGRESS CATALOGING-IN-PUBLICATION DATA:
Kelly, Kate.
Living safe in an unsafe world : the complete guide to family preparedness /
Kate Kelly ; with an introduction by Randall C. Duncan.
p.    cm.
Includes index.
ISBN 0-451-40932-9
1. Accidents—Prevention.    2. Home accidents—Prevention.
3. Crime prevention.    4. Wounds and injuries—Prevention.    I. Title.
HV675   .K398   2000
613.6—dc21
00-037246

PUBLISHER'S NOTE
Every effort has been made to ensure that the information contained in this book is complete and accurate. However, each emergency situation presents unique issues and problems. Thus the ideas, procedures, and suggestions in this book must be viewed in context and considered in light of your own good judgment. This book is not intended as a substitute for consulting with your physician and obtaining medical supervision as to any activity, procedure, or suggestion that might affect your health or the health of your child. Accordingly, individual readers must assume responsibility for their own actions, safety, and health and neither the author nor the publisher shall be liable or responsible for any loss, injury, or damage allegedly arising from any information or suggestion in this book.

*To George, who has always made certain our family
has been prepared for anything.*

# Acknowledgments

This book could not have been written without the aid of many people, three of whom provided a wealth of information to me on a recurring basis. Emergency Manager Randall C. Duncan, who has provided an intelligent "must read" introduction for the book, has made himself available to me throughout the preparation of the book, to offer insight on a wide variety of subjects and to help put some of the advice in perspective so that it was clear what actions should take priority. His advice has been consistently realistic as to what safety measures were practical, and which were just extra work for families, and I am deeply grateful for his contributions to the book.

Rocky Lopes, Ph.D., of the American Red Cross, has also been available for questions at all times, and he willingly read through the 550-page manuscript in the heat of the summer, all to be certain that readers would be getting the most accurate and up-to-date preparedness information that is available. Rocky Lopes also worked with the National Disaster Education Coalition in writing *Talking About Disasters: Guide for Standard Messages* (May 1999), a public service publication upon which some of the natural disaster content was based.

Researcher Bernadette Sukley's well-organized investigations into so many topics were key to making the book comprehensive in scope, and the book benefited from her research skills as well as her intelligence and past experience in writing about issues concerning health and safety.

In addition to these three key people, there were specialists and organization representatives who answered questions, sent me material, and pointed me toward helpful websites. I am indebted to the following for tolerating continual phone calls: To Kevin Brenner of Brenner Builders for explaining to me how to keep houses standing and in working order, regardless of what happens; to Kathryn Creedy of the Federal Aviation Administration, who talked me through every type of safety measure to take when a family travels by air; to Warren Flatou of the Federal Railroad Administration, who took time to help me navigate my way to information regarding rail safety; to Jill Fredston of the Alaska Mountain Safety Center, who gave advice on both avalanches and bears; to Garrett Graaskamp of the Office of Ground Water and Drinking Water, who was willing to answer countless questions about all types of water safety; to Peggy Glenn, who long ago made me aware of the importance of fire safety; to Terri Harris of the National Self Defense Institute, who gave unstintingly of her time in discussing personal safety with me; to Lynn Landes of Zero Waste America, who opened my eyes regarding the unsafe world we're creating through poor waste management; to Jean Salvatore of the Insurance Information Institute, who knew the answers to all my insurance questions; to Sue Snider, Ph.D., a food and nutrition expert with the University of Delaware who was one among several food safety experts who were particularly helpful in providing information about safe foods; to Rick Yates, a ranger with the Glacier National Park, who was helpful in updating the information regarding newly observed aggression in bears. Allergy expert Dr. William Storms was one of many medical professionals who were willing to fill me in on details on a wide variety of subjects. In addition, I received first-rate information from countless organizations ranging from the Humane Society of the United States to the Center for the Prevention of

School Violence and the National School Safety Center; from the Chicago Herpetological Society and Florida's Fish and Wildlife Conservation Commission to the railroad's Operation Lifesaver. It took files and files to keep track of all the research for this book, and I am grateful to all who helped provide me with such fascinating reading.

This book had to have a beginning, and the fact that I was considered as the writer is due to agent Liza Dawson, who called me when she heard that NAL was looking for someone to write a family preparedness guide. Liza also provided first-rate advice whenever I needed it.

Ellen Edwards, my editor on this project, has been a dream to work with. Her instinct as to what topics should be included was nothing short of prescient, and her attention to the manuscript has made it a much better book. Thank you, Ellen.

—Kate Kelly
January 2000

# Contents

# A Personal Note from the Author

"Ah, a book for the paranoid," was a comment made again and again when I described to people the book I was researching and writing.

Not at all, I've discovered. *Living Safe in an Unsafe World: The Complete Guide to Family Preparedness* is a book for us all, because there's not a parent I know who doesn't place a priority on keeping his or her family safe.

While I've always been casually safety conscious, particularly when it came to my children, I never worried for a moment about things I hadn't experienced. I never considered how to get out of a multistory hotel in case of fire, or gave any thought to what I would do if I was visiting my brother in the Midwest when a tornado touched down. Car jacking? That was something that happened to somebody else. "Airplane rage"? I'd read about it but never experienced it.

Now I know what a mistake I've made, barely in time to rectify it and share what I've learned with my growing children.

As I researched topic after topic for this book, one message came through to me from all sources. The more you know about a potential danger, the less frightening it becomes, and the more you gain a sense of confidence about your ability to handle it.

"Aren't you totally freaked out by thinking about all those disasters?" was another question I was asked, and I can honestly say, "Not at all. I enjoyed it." While I will readily admit to still feeling uneasy about a few of the subjects I address in the book, for the most part, the information I learned has given me a tremendous sense of calm. I now know what to do in many situations that could befall any one of us, and I have gained a fair degree of assurance that I could deal with most of them.

My current project is educating my children, a "favor" they don't always appreciate. As they run off to school, the beach, or a hiking trip, I arm them with facts about what preventive measures they need to take to stay safe.

I sincerely hope the information imparted in this book will bring you the feeling of control that it has brought me. May we as parents collectively work to make safety a matter of course for our children. Then maybe they won't panic if they're approached by a ferocious dog or if they're at an amusement park when lightning strikes. They'll know what to do because they were brought up to make "safety" a part of their lives.

# How to Use this Book

You might start by reading Certified Emergency Manager Randall C. Duncan's introductory comments. He provides several important points for anyone who is concerned about safety. You might also give his "situational awareness" exercise a try.

Next, I suggest you need to read Chapters 1–5, where you'll learn about the mental mind-set that will help you put safety first. You'll gain some special emergency guidelines and get a complete blueprint for preparing your Family Disaster Plan. These early chapters will also provide you with a list of important supplies to keep on hand and some vital information about how to make certain you have enough insurance coverage.

After you've covered those basics, let your level of interest be your guide, and read about whatever you want—from killer bees to volcanic eruptions. The most important chapters, however, may not be the most enticing: Car accidents still cause almost half of all accidental deaths in this country. I urge you to take a moment to go through the chapters concerning car safety. There's some great information about "road rage," something that affects all of us. Look, too, at the chapter on safety restraints. The injury and death statistics will improve if more people use restraint systems properly.

As you go through the book, you may wonder why I include

certain subjects and not others. I used two criterion for inclusion: The first was the "worry" factor. Even if it wasn't a statistically alarming problem, were people worried about it? Although "Mad Cow Disease" is not a widespread illness, it has been in the news a great deal. For that reason, I wanted readers to fully understand what the disease is, whether they need to be concerned, and how to protect their family.

My second criterion for including certain topics concerned alarming statistics. For example, although a great deal has already been written about the damage done to our skin by the sun, the statistics for skin cancer remain quite sobering. I wanted readers to have the latest data on a subject that obviously still needs our attention.

## HIGHLIGHTED INFORMATION

As you read through the chapters in Part Two, you'll note that each section includes "Top Tips to Teach Your Children" as well as summary information under a "Hot Button" heading. My purpose in highlighting this information is to make the preparedness process as easy as possible. For example, the section concerning earthquakes is extremely long, but what your children need to remember can be reduced to a couple of essential tips: They need to understand the part of the family disaster plan that pertains to them, and they ought to know (and be drilled in) "Drop, Cover, and Hold on."

The "Hot Button" information serves a similar purpose. If you remember only the three or four summary points about flash floods, snake bites, or a chemical accident, you'll be well-enough prepared to use common sense to survive.

I hope the book will serve as a handy reference volume that also makes for interesting reading. The world is sometimes a dangerous place, but with this book you'll have the information you need to keep you and your family safe—no matter what happens.

—Kate Kelly

# Certified Emergency Manager Randall C. Duncan Addresses Family Safety

Living and working in Wichita, Kansas, right in Tornado Alley, I am constantly amazed at people who have been longtime residents yet choose to ignore the obvious clues Mother Nature gives during a severe weather season. As the Sedgwick County Director of Emergency Management, I frequently give severe weather awareness talks to neighborhood associations and other groups. The primary caution I give, the one they most need to hear, is, "If you walk outside and it's a muggy, hot, overcast afternoon in Kansas and the sky is pea soup green, and there's a feeling in the air that makes the little hairs on the back of your neck stand up, that's Mother Nature telling you there's a storm coming. Please pay attention."

This is certainly Lesson One in coping with any emergency. Sometimes in our highly modernized life we shut out the signals our forefathers relied upon to keep them safe. There will never be a day when we can afford to ignore the clues around us.

In my position as an emergency manager, I have seen how people react in all kinds of desperate situations. Those who run into serious problems tend to be the ones who don't take the time to think.

To get started on making your family better prepared for living safely in an unsafe world, there are three lessons I'd like you to focus on right from the beginning:

## 1. BUILD "SITUATIONAL AWARENESS"

While some dangers and disasters can be prevented or minimized with proper precautions, there are many times when the unexpected occurs. A tornado hits all of a sudden. A "road rage" driver starts tailing you dangerously on the highway. You can't control whether or not you encounter these experiences; what you can control is your reaction to them.

Responding well in such situations is a *developed* talent, not something you're born with. Even if you're a person who tends to panic when confronted with an emergency, you can learn to react in a more helpful manner by developing what I call "situational awareness."

Some people are already very good at taking in their surroundings and adjusting their behavior to fit what is happening around them—even in stressful situations. This makes them more likely to respond appropriately.

You can actually improve the way you respond to emergencies by working to achieve greater situational awareness. Try this exercise one day when you're driving on the highway:

*Imagine you're driving along listening to your favorite radio station, and thinking about all you have to do the next day. Suddenly you blow a tire or are forced off the road by another driver. You have your cell phone with you. Will you be able to describe to emergency personnel where you are and direct them to within a mile of your location?*

If you answer yes, then you're almost certainly the type of person who will be an asset when confronted with an emergency.

If you're not certain whether you could describe your location to emergency personnel, then start practicing—it's a learnable skill. Whenever you're in the car, practice identifying where you are. As you become more observant, you'll find your level of "situational awareness" increasing. This skill will spill over into other types of circumstances in which your ability to assess what's happening will be key. For example, mentally review what you would do in a variety of the situations that are described in this book:

- You're on vacation and it's a beautiful day, but when you show up at the tennis courts, there's a notice posted about the hurricane that's been making the news: "Instructions to visitors and residents: Evacuate immediately." What would you do next?
- Your child is playing in the backyard one afternoon when a raccoon wanders on to your property. What should you do?
- You're in an airplane that has just taken off and the pilot announces you're circling back around for an emergency landing. How should you prepare?
- Your college-age daughter has just called to say she woke up and found a bat in her dorm room. What should you tell her?

The art to managing each of these situations lies in remaining calm, taking into account all that is happening, and one additional ingredient—the second point I'd like you to remember:

## 2. ALWAYS USE COMMON SENSE

When faced with any unexpected situation—from a threatening dog to a major storm—the person who manages well will be the one who takes a deep breath, considers the situation, and then employs good old-fashioned common sense in determining how best to assure a positive outcome.

During the 1998–99 school year, a Ball State college student was driving on a road in the vicinity of Muncie, Indiana, where Ball State is located. Visibility was reduced by poor weather conditions and somehow her car encountered a train and got hooked on to it. There must have been little impact from the collision because the engineer proceeded along his route, unaware that he had a car and young driver in tow. Using the cell phone she had with her in the car, the student had the common sense and presence of mind to phone her mother. Emergency personnel were able to respond more quickly because of her call, and she almost certainly saved her own life because she kept her head and used good sense in handling the emergency. The only thing she might have done better was to have called 9-1-1 first, but we've all got moms—we understand why she called her first.

Whenever you're confronted with a dangerous situation, take a deep breath and quickly look for the best—or at least a logical— solution. Whether you're facing a flooding roadway or helping a child who has just been bitten by a snake, you'll find that common sense will tide you through until trained personnel arrive to help.

## 3. PRACTICE

What makes the final difference? Practice.

Have you ever heard the saying, "You play like you practice"? There's no doubt that we do the things we're trained to do. In this book you'll read about family fire drills, earthquake drills, and tornado drills as well as what to do if heatstroke or frostbite threatens. Plan out these drills and practice them with your children. Reading about these situations is good; practicing them is better.

Detailed advice on coping with and surviving specific unsafe conditions follows in this book and will give you the knowledge you need to protect you and your family. In the meantime, if you develop a heightened sense of situational awareness, employ common sense, and practice some of the emergency drills; you'll already be a step ahead of everyone else in handling an emergency.

—Randall C. Duncan, Certified Emergency Manager
Director, Sedgwick County Emergency Management
Member and Immediate Past-president,
International Association of Emergency Managers

# PART ONE

# GENERAL FAMILY PREPAREDNESS

## Chapter 1

# Simple Steps Families
# Can Take to Prepare

Every day you can pick up the newspaper and read about a new disaster that has occurred in some part of the country. If you include the international news, the number of dangers you could worry about becomes virtually limitless.

While the media may present the world as an extremely perilous place, there's no reason to panic. According to *American Demographics* magazine, accidental injury rates are at an all-time low. Though mishaps still kill one American every six minutes, the drop in accident rates proves that safety education and preparedness do help.

This book is intended to make you aware of what can happen and to provide you with a plan that will get you through any emergency.

## SEVEN SIMPLE STEPS TO SPEED YOUR EMERGENCY RESPONSE

While carrying out a safety plan during a tornado is quite different from responding to a fire, there are some emergency preparation basics that are easy to do. Read through the following

list, and even if this is all you can do for now, you will have taken
an important step toward taking good care of your family.

**1. *Develop "situational awareness."*** The first step in responding well in an emergency is learning to spot one early
enough to cope intelligently with it. You can avoid being part of a
multicar pile up on the highway if your advance road-scanning
(a technique described later in the book) tells you there's a
problem up ahead. Or you can get out of an angry crowd before
it becomes riotous if you're paying attention to the signals. In
his introduction, Sedgwick (Kansas) County Emergency Manager Randy Duncan explains the importance of situational awareness and provides an exercise to help you heighten your own
awareness.

**2. *Drill into your head your main priority: life before
property.*** Although the training you've had to "hold on to your
stuff" may lead you to grab your purse or briefcase even when exiting a plane in an emergency, you've got to fight that instinct.
The seconds it takes to reach for a possession may be seconds
you can't afford; they may make the difference between life and
death. Newspaper reports and television news frequently describe tragedies that befall people who run back into a burning home to save a family photo album or who decide to stay
home during a hurricane to "protect" their possessions. In a life-
threatening situation, there's only one decision to make: Save
yourself and those around you. Only if there is time should you
consider saving your property.

**3. *Get training.*** Take an American Red Cross first aid and
CPR course to learn how to treat burns and cuts and how to give
rescue breathing and administer CPR.

**4. *Equip your home with fire extinguishers and learn
how to use them.*** In countless situations, fire is a byproduct of
another disaster. In the 1906 San Francisco earthquake, the resulting fires caused more damage than the earthquake itself. And
while phoning "9-1-1" should be your first response when you

spot fire or smell smoke, using a fire extinguisher is appropriate in some situations.

**5.** *Learn how to shut off your utilities.* Earthquakes, fires, storms, and floods can all damage utility lines, causing gas leaks, electrical fires, and broken water mains. You may need to turn off your utilities to save lives and property, so if you don't already know how to do this, turn to the Appendix and learn how now.

**6.** *Take an active role in your community's prepared-ness planning.* In Jackson, Tennessee, in January of 1999, eight of the city's 20 sirens weren't working when a tornado hit. Even with easy access to radio, television, and storm watches over the Internet, it's important for communities to maintain their warn-ing systems so that as many people as possible can be notified in the event of an emergency.

**7.** *Think of your neighbors.* When there is a local emer-gency, think of the elderly couple across the street who may need help. And think of your neighbors in a global sense, too. In the summer of 1999, when the northeast was suffering a terrible drought, there were still people who felt they had the right to wa-ter their lawns each day. This was particularly galling in New Jer-sey, where some people still irrigated even after the governor placed water restrictions on local residents. And in Hurricane Floyd (also in 1999), emergency managers realized that one rea-son the highways were so crowded during evacuation of the southeastern coastal states was because families loaded up and took as many vehicles as they had drivers. Rather than "elbowing others out of the way" in a time of crisis by putting more value on your own property than on the lives of other people, try to think of how you can extend a helping hand. Someday someone may do the same for you or a family member.

## THE IMPORTANCE OF WARNING SIGNS

*Pay attention to warnings.* In situations ranging from the shootings at Columbine High School in Littleton, Colorado, to the bombing at the U.S. Embassy in Nairobi, there were intimations that something was going to happen. Something about the situation had become uncomfortable enough to suggest to more than one person that trouble was brewing. If you sense that something isn't right, or if you hear a specific threat, pay attention to it. Your gut instinct can be a powerful tool in your own defense.

*As soon as you sense an emergency, react.* Because we're not accustomed to dealing with disasters or crises (and perhaps because of a certain numbness fostered by the violence we witness on television), there is a tendency for people to "sit there" waiting to see if what is happening is real. Move quickly. Find out later that your precautions were not needed after all. Fewer people would have been hurt in accidents ranging from fires to rock concert stampedes if people had responded at the first signs of danger. Even if you discover later that it was a false alarm, don't take a chance by not reacting.

## SIX WAYS TO HELP YOUR CHILDREN PREPARE

"I don't want to scare them," you may be thinking. Many parents feel that way, little realizing that there is a way to make children take safety and emergency preparedness in stride:

**1. *Make safety issues a routine part of family life.*** Whether it's slathering on sunscreen each day (including cloudy days), learning to approach other people's pets cautiously, or counting the rows on a plane between your family's seats and the emergency exits, you can establish a pattern of preparedness that seems totally natural to your child. Explain to them that when people know what to do in an emergency, it makes the situation much easier to handle.

**2. *Teach children how and when to call for help.*** If your community is not part of the 9-1-1 emergency response system, then help your child memorize the number they should dial in an emergency. (Post these numbers as well.)

**3. *Make sure everyone in the family knows the name of the county you live in.*** Much emergency information is dispensed on a county-wide basis, and it's never too early for children to understand what pertains to them and what doesn't. When you travel, find out what county you're visiting, and share that information with the kids. In Louisiana, emergency information is announced by parish; in Alaska, it's by borough.

**4. *Practice responding to emergencies with your children.*** With little ones, you can make it a game: "Where do we go in a fire? Let's do it!" "Where do we go in a tornado? Let's do it!" "What should we do if a scary dog comes toward us?"

While you wouldn't want to run a sequence of these "drills" all on one day, you can make a family activity of asking questions like this out of the blue. You'll soon find your child will get an "A" in emergency preparedness!

**5. *Encourage older children to take a first aid course.*** These are critical skills and will be helpful to them throughout life. (Baby-sitters who have first aid training can charge more, so you can offer that as an additional incentive.)

**6. *Teach your children to take emergencies seriously. They can't afford to assume everything is "just another school fire drill."*** Ignoring a school fire-alarm bell during an after-school activity or not responding to an emergency warning in a museum is a big mistake. Children, especially teens, sometimes feel: "It won't happen to me," but they need to be raised with a healthy respect for the fact that it most certainly could happen to them. They'll be just fine if they know what to do.

# Chapter 2

# Emergencies: Getting Organized

"Now, where did I put that?" are the wrong words to have to utter in the midst of an emergency. Whether you're phoning your pediatrician to ask about a rash or you need to remember where your "emergency papers" are before you evacuate during a flood, organization will bring you peace of mind.

## CREATE AN EMERGENCY NOTEBOOK

- Purchase a standard-size loose-leaf notebook, 8½ x 11 lined paper, and subject dividers with pockets that will let you create categories within the notebook.
- The first page in the notebook should be the emergency telephone numbers you have posted by the phone. Add the phone numbers of any friends or relatives you might want to contact in a prolonged emergency. (See the section concerning "On-the-Go Emergency Listings.")
- Your notebook should be tailored to your exact needs. Depending on the area of the country in which you live, certain subjects will be relevant and others won't. While

everyone should have an "In case of Fire" category, those who live in a hurricane-prone area should create a separate category that explains your family plan in case of a hurricane.

- Also create a "Home Emergencies" category for what to do in certain household emergencies:

  - what needs to be turned off if the basement floods
  - who should be called if the power goes out
  - list the names and telephone numbers of your plumber and electrician as well as any other person who knows your house well and could help you cope with an emergency

- Set aside a page with a diagram or written instructions showing how to turn off your power, gas, and water. Everyone thinks they'll remember this information, but you may not need it for years. By that time you may have forgotten, and directions or a diagram to follow will be very handy.
- Also use the notebook to keep track of other information that concerns you. For example, in many parts of the country, Lyme disease is a current concern. Use the pocket dividers to keep helpful articles on the topic. The notebook pages can be used to record the name and number of a specialist or the date and any additional information about a family member who has exhibited symptoms.

## EMERGENCY TELEPHONE NUMBERS

Make one emergency list to be photocopied and posted at your main telephones upstairs and downstairs. Note numbers for:

Fire _____

Police _____

Poison Control Center _____

Ambulance _____

Electric company emergency number _____

Gas company emergency number _____

Pediatrician _____

Pediatric Dentist _____

Pharmacy _____

Veterinarian _____


Work Numbers—Mother _____

Father _____

Neighbor who would help _____

In-town relative to notify _____

Out-of-town Emergency Contact _____

Taxi _____

Nearest hospital and address _____

_____

Each child's name, birth date, and blood type:

_____

_____


## CREATE ON-THE-GO EMERGENCY LISTINGS

When faced with a crisis, many of us may cope well enough on a moment-to-moment basis, but our ability to retrieve simple information may be affected by the anxiety we're feeling. We might suddenly be hard-pressed to remember our own phone number. For this reason, the sensible thing is to create several "emergency number" directories that can go where you go or be kept in helpful places like the glove compartment of the car. Plan to have one of these directories in each of the family cars as well as one to store with your important papers, the ones you'll take with you in an emergency.

- Buy the number of blank pocket directories you think you'll need.
- List in each the names, birth dates, and blood types of all family members as well as any special medical conditions or information you might need to provide in an emergency. (For example, the name of the surgical procedure your daughter underwent two years ago—something you know now, but might forget under stress.) Writing down things you already know may seem like a waste of time, but you'll find that doing so brings a degree of calm. In an emergency, you'll find that there's one less thing you have to think about; you can simply open the directory and read what a physician would need to know.
- List all phone numbers you might need in an emergency. The list you've posted by your telephone is a good start, but if you had to evacuate your home for a few days, there are probably more names and numbers you would like to have with you. Give yourself a few days to think about who else should be listed in these directories.
- Write down anything else you think you might forget under stress.
- Fill out each directory and put it in the appropriate car or with your important papers. (If your telephone directory is computerized, this process may be as simple as printing out a selective version of the directory a few times.)

## SELECT A SECURE HOLDING PLACE FOR CASH AND PAPERS

Important papers—including identification for all members of the family—and cash are absolutely necessary to help get you through certain emergencies, and since there may not be time to hunt down the papers you need or run to the ATM, the best thing to do is to select a secret spot for keeping these things. You may only feel comfortable if these items are tucked in a home safe, or you may be perfectly happy stashing them under a pile of clothing in the attic. Keep in mind that you or your spouse should have access to this material, so designate a spot on which you both agree. Be sure to tell the other person if for some reason the items must be moved.

- Here are the family documents you'll want to gather:

  - ◆ Record of bank accounts.
  - ◆ Family record (copies of birth, marriage, death certificates).
  - ◆ Inventory of valuable household goods (See Chapter Five "Insuring Against Disaster").
  - ◆ Copies of will, insurance policies, contracts, deeds, stocks and bonds.
  - ◆ Record of credit card account numbers and companies.
  - ◆ Copy of passports, social security cards, immunization records.

- Make three copies of the above, giving you a total of four copies:

  1. Store the originals of these papers in a safe deposit box.
  2. One of the copies should be stored in a file cabinet in your home, partly because this provides ready reference when you want to check to see what you have.
  3. One copy should be in this secret spot where you can grab the papers and cash at a moment's notice.
  4. Send the other copies to your out-of-the-area emergency contact. If you have to leave home without grabbing these documents, you can get what you need at your bank safe deposit box or by calling your emergency contact.

- Cash. Plan to keep about two weeks' worth of spending money in your home. Emergency managers in the 1994 Northridge, California, earthquake found that one of the biggest problems was people's lack of money—banks were closed and access to ATMs was denied for a period of time.

If a crisis is such that you can get out of the area, you'll be able to use a credit card elsewhere until you can regain access to your bank. However, in a regional disaster where evacuation isn't practical or possible, it will be handy to have cash readily available.

Some families will feel more comfortable if this money is hidden in two or three places so that if a thief finds one place, the entire stash won't necessarily be stolen.

To feel secure about these measures, it's essential that you don't discuss them widely. If you're unaccustomed to keeping large sums of money around the house, there will be no reason for someone to think you are now, unless you talk about it.

## IN CASE OF EMERGENCY: PREPARATIONS FOR A BABY-SITTER

- Show any caregiver you hire the notebook, and explain to her the appropriate safety measures you would expect her to take if anything were to happen.
- Prepare an emergency envelope, and leave it in a designated spot. It should contain:

    - Emergency money (for cab fare, gas, etc.). Include change for the telephone, at least four quarters and four dimes (if the public phone in your town charges 35 cents).
    - Extra copy of your emergency numbers.
    - Two index cards with clear instructions:

        1. Name of hospital, phone number, exactly how to get there, and location of the emergency entrance.
        2. Pediatrician's name, address, phone number, and directions to the office.

- ◆ Emergency consent form, leaving your most often used sitter as the designated person in charge. (See following sample.)
- ◆ Also include a card with information on each child:

Name _____

Birth date _____ Blood Type _____

Date of last tetanus toxoid shot _____

Allergies (particularly any to medication): _____

_____

Chronic or past illnesses: _____

_____

Health Insurance Company and ID # _____

_____

- • Review the contents of the envelope with any new caregiver or evening baby-sitter. In an emergency, instruct her to take the entire envelope with her.
- • Make a copy of all material in the emergency envelope to create a second envelope to keep in the diaper bag at all times. Should an emergency occur at the playground, you or your caregiver would have all the information necessary.
- • Show your caregiver your Emergency Notebook, and point out to her any pages that you think might be particularly relevant.

## EMERGENCY CONSENT FORM

In case you cannot be reached, the person who is caring for your children should have a notarized letter from you giving over temporary medical authority. Prepare one for your mother if she's in charge for a weekend; give one to your nanny if you work outside the house. The following sample may not be legal in all states. Consult an attorney, or ask your pediatrician for a form that would work in your state.

## AUTHORIZATION FOR EMERGENCY MEDICAL CARE

Date _____

Child _____

In the event that my child needs immediate medical attention and we cannot be reached, I/we give authority to _____

_____

to request appropriate medical care for our child. If our regular pediatrician is unavailable, then the pediatrician on duty at the hospital may provide or obtain medical care for my child.

Signed _____
(mother)

Signed _____
(father)

Mother _____   Phone _____
Father _____   Phone _____
Pediatrician _____   Phone _____

Notary signature _____

- If your child has a health problem and regularly sees more than one physician, list those names and numbers as well.
- Because the letter needs to be notarized, do this in advance, especially if you're going out of town.

# Chapter 3

# Create a Disaster Plan for Your Family

Uncertainty and chaos are big problems during an emergency. Initially, our first worries concern the whereabouts of family members: "Should I try to go and find her? What if she's on her way to find me?"

That's why you need to plan. Spending the time now to consider what you and your family would do in a crisis will bring you clarity of mind in a true emergency.

## INFORMATION IS KEY

There are some important safety habits to instill in family members well in advance of an emergency:

- All family members should always wear or have identification on them. (If anyone is injured badly and alone, you will want that person to be "labeled," so you've got to get family members in the habit of wearing ID now.) When children are little, using identification on their sneakers is highly practical as most kids wear play shoes most of the time. As they get older, you need to work with them on what makes sense based on their lifestyle. A cloth name tape (sold as camp clothing labels) in a few often worn articles of clothing may accomplish what you need. As the kids get older, teach them to make a point of slipping on, or pinning to themselves, something with their name in it before they go out. Any family member with special medical issues can also note those on any type of ID.

Seasonally evaluate your children's wardrobe changes and see which articles of clothing can easily be labeled.

- Impress on children the importance of checking in, and require them to do it as a matter of course. Your eleven-year-old should call when he and his bike buddies have moved to someone else's house to play, and your 17-year-old should check in as well when her plans change. This type of automatic response is key in an emergency. If your children aren't with you, you want them to immediately think of calling you or your designated emergency contact.
- Once they go to college, stress that you would like to hear from them if there are unusual circumstances. For example, if news reports describe your child's college town as "devastated by a hurricane," tell him or her that it's important to contact you to say, "Hey, it's a mess here, but I'm okay."

## RESEARCH AND PLANNING

- Find out what disaster plans are in effect at your workplace, your children's school or day care center, and any other places where members of your family spend time. Understanding what may happen if you're all elsewhere during the day will be important in developing contingency plans.
- Stock up on emergency supplies, and assemble a Disaster Supples Kit (see next chapter). Once it's organized, select a convenient place for it (perhaps the bottom or back of a closet—nearby but not in the way). Be sure everyone knows where it is.

- Make a list of what you would take with you if you were told you had five minutes to pack before you had to leave your house. If there were news of a flood or fire in your area, you wouldn't even have to think before knowing what items to put in your car trunk in case of evacuation. Then if you are told to leave, you can do so quickly because you are well organized.
- Plan what you would do if you have to evacuate. Call your local American Red Cross chapter or the emergency management office in your area to find out what would happen if your community had to evacuate. Based on this information, select an alternate evacuation route, and make copies of your plan along with a copy of an area map. Put one in the Emergency Notebook and one in each of your cars.

## PLACES AND CONTACTS

- Prearrange two family meeting spots. Give each a name— even a funny one—so that you'll have a way to differentiate between them.

  - *Pick one spot near your home:* This spot is where the family would meet if you had to leave the house (such as in a fire) or if you could get to the neighborhood but not into your house. This is the "nose counting" location to make certain that everyone at home has emerged safely. Some people designate a tree or a fence post as a meeting place, but it is preferable to select the home of a nearby neighbor. If one family member is out of the area, it provides a way for the person to check in on the whereabouts of the rest of the family.
  - *The other spot should be outside your neighborhood:* Again, it is preferable to select a person's home as your "away from home" meeting spot so that family members

who can't reach the area as quickly as you might like can phone.

All family members should know the names, addresses, and phone numbers of the meeting locations.

◆ *Designate an emergency phone contact:* a family member or a friend—who lives far enough away not to be caught in the same disaster. This person could be in another county or different state. If some of you are at work or at school when a disaster hits, try to leave a message as to your whereabouts as soon as possible so that this person can begin to keep track of where everyone is. During a disaster, local calls on hard-wired telephones may be difficult to make, but it may be possible to make long-distance calls. Cell phones sometimes don't work in community-wide disasters.

◆ *Give relatives the name and number of your designated contact:* That way they can call the designee for information about where you are and how everyone is doing.

◆ *Help children memorize names and telephone numbers they might need in an emergency:* (If they've taken cover at a neighbor's house during a tornado and can't get through to you, they should have no doubt about who they are to call next.)

## ESTABLISH SIMPLE FAMILY RESPONSE PLANS FOR EMERGENCIES

Every family should have a "Fire Response" plan, but your other emergency plans will depend on where you live. Californians will want to write out what to do in an earthquake; Oklahomans will make particular note of tornadoes. If you're in an area where there are frequent brushfires, you'll want to have a plan for that type of emergency. As you read this book, you'll learn how different disasters require different responses.

After reading the relevant sections of the book and making

some basic decisions for your family, put this information in your Emergency Notebook, and keep it in a central location such as the kitchen. Hold a family meeting to discuss the plans.

- In some emergencies, your safest place is right at home. Select locations for where you would wait out various types of emergencies. Any child old enough to stay at home alone should understand the difference between what to do in a fire and what to do in a tornado. (In a tornado he should go to the lowest interior point in the house and cover his head to protect against falling debris; in a fire, he should get out of the house as quickly as possible.)
- Have a plan and contingency plans. Spell out different steps to take based on where you might be—home, school, work, in the yard, or in a car. Despite the complexity of having to create more than one plan, try to keep each very simple, so that it's easy to remember in a crisis. Keep everything as consistent as possible. For example, if you're in charge of picking up your toddler in case of a crisis, try to always be the parent in charge of that child so your child will know exactly who to expect.
- Be very explicit with family members about what will happen in an emergency if they are not with you. Discuss what the emergency plan is for their school or workplace, and explain who will try to go get whom and why it's important to wait in a designated place.
- Update these plans each school year in case there have been changes.

## ADDITIONAL SAFETY INFORMATION TO KNOW

- As early as possible, teach your children about calling 9-1-1 in an emergency. There have been countless times when children have made crucial calls.

- *If the 9-1-1 system ever goes down, dial "0" for the operator and ask to be put through to emergency personnel.* Operators can find alternative lines if the 9-1-1 system is not functioning.
- If someone requires medical attention, call 9-1-1 and ask that medical help be sent; don't plan to drive to the hospital yourself. The response team will have been trained to make an initial evaluation and to start emergency procedures if necessary. In disaster situations, roads may be blocked by law enforcement officials. The only way to get a person to a hospital would be by an emergency response vehicle.
- The American Red Cross strongly recommends that everyone take a first aid course so that they can provide immediate care for anyone who is injured until medical help can arrive.

## CREATING A DISASTER PLAN FOR YOUR PETS

If your family is like most families with pets, the crying and moaning over the possibility of leaving Rover or Fluffy behind will slow the process of responding to an emergency. For that reason, the best thing you can do for your family—and your pets—is to create an emergency plan for them as well.

- Make sure your pet has some form of ID on the collar, that includes your name and number. At least 1.6 million American pets now have "identification" microchips embedded under their skin to make it easier to determine who the animal is and to whom it belongs.
- If you must evacuate, try to take the animals to a safe place. Pets are not allowed in public shelters or in those operated by the Red Cross, so if there is any chance that a shelter would be your family's destination, you'll need to make other plans for your pets. Research in advance what your options might be:

◆ Ask friends or relatives. One of these individuals should be located in a different community. If your town floods, any in-town family will have the same problem you will.

◆ Contact hotels and motels ouside your immediate area and ask about their policies on accepting pets. Keep a list of "pet friendly" places in your Emergency Notebook and in your on-the-go telephone directories.

◆ Prepare a list of boarding facilities and veterinarians who could shelter animals in an emergency—try to get 24-hour telephone numbers, and list these as well.

● In the event that you're not home at the time of a crisis or an evacuation, make arrangements with a neighbor who would be willing to bring your pets to an agreed-upon place.

### If a disaster is approaching:

● Bring your pets in so that you won't have to search for them if you have to leave in a hurry. If your cat is prone to hiding when stressed, put her in a carrier as soon as you sense there may be a problem.

● Call ahead to reserve or confirm a place to stay with relatives, friends, or at a pet friendly hotel.

● If there is time, fasten adhesive tape onto the ID with the telephone number of where your pet will be staying written on it.

● Pets under stress may not react normally. Keep dogs leashed and cats in carriers. Don't give them an opportunity to escape. Losing them elsewhere would be yet another very unfortunate consequence of a disaster.

### If you absolutely can't bring your animal with you:

● Make certain your pet is wearing a collar with ID.

● Post a notice on your door about the fact that pets are inside and that the animal control people should be called. Leave a phone number as well.

- Confine your pet to an interior room that has ventilation but no windows. Leave them with several days supply of dry food and a bathtub full or several buckets of water—animals drink a lot when under stress.
- Don't leave animals together unless they are well-matched.

# Chapter 4

# Your Disaster Supplies Kit(s)

Whether a broken water main has caused officials to turn off the water in your town, a winter storm has snowbound your entire family for a weekend, or a hurricane has forced you to evacuate, it's important to have a reasonable quantity of special supplies on hand. This chapter lists what you will need as well as when you might need it.

However, before putting together your basic supplies, consider the following:

## TWO ITEMS WORTH THE INVESTMENT

**1. *A cellular phone:*** Countless crises and emergencies can be made more manageable with a cellular telephone. If you don't currently own one, it's worth the investment for emergency purposes. Whether your car breaks down at night or your household catches fire, a cell phone can be invaluable. What's more, by 2001 the Federal Communications Commission will require cellular phone companies to have the technology in place to be able to provide 9-1-1 operators with the location of anyone calling on a cell phone so that help can get to the right place as quickly as possible.

**2. *NOAA Weather Radio:*** A National Oceanic and Atmospheric Administration weather radio is also worth the money. (Eventually they'll be as prevalent as smoke alarms.) The National Weather Service continuously broadcasts updated weather warnings and forecasts that can be received by NOAA Weather Radios, and they now broadcast warnings and post-event information for all types of hazards. Because it is tied into the Emergency Alert System, the NOAA Weather Radio can be considered an "all hazards" radio network, making it the single best source of emergency information. The National Weather Service recommends buying one that has both a battery backup and a Specific Area Message Encoder (SAME) feature, which automatically alerts you when a watch or warning is issued for your county. The National Weather Radio signal is a line-of-sight signal, which does not bore through hills or mountains.

## PREPARING THE "BASICS" KIT

- These basic items might be useful at home in an emergency, but the list also provides you with "starter" items in the event of an evacuation:

  - A portable, battery-powered radio (preferably NOAA) and extra batteries
  - Flashlight and extra batteries
  - First aid kit (see below) with first aid manual
  - Supply of prescription medications (Check with your pharmacist or physician about how best to store any of the medicines you're putting away for an emergency; you may need to replace them periodically.)
  - Credit card and cash
  - Personal identification for you and other members of the family

- ◆ Extra set of car keys
- ◆ Matches in a waterproof container
- ◆ Map of the area
- ◆ Your on-the-go phone directory
- ◆ Special needs such as diapers or formula for an infant, extra glasses or hearing aid batteries for those who need them.

- Store these items in a backpack or duffel bag that you keep near an exit, such as in the bottom of the entry hall closet.
- Make certain all family members know where the "Basics" duffel is kept.
- An emergency supplies kit with slightly different contents should be placed in the back of each car that you own. A complete list of supplies for your car is listed in the "Car Safety" section with additional winter supplies mentioned in "Winter Storms."

*At home you may need:* A wrench to turn off the household gas and water. Keep it near the shutoff valves. (See the Appendix for more information.)

## FIRST AID KIT

- In a separate small bag, pack the following medical items:

  - ◆ first aid manual
  - ◆ sterile adhesive bandages, gauze pads and rolls
  - ◆ scissors
  - ◆ hypoallergenic adhesive tape
  - ◆ hydrogen peroxide
  - ◆ pain reliever and antacid tablets
  - ◆ snakebite kit
  - ◆ tweezers

- ◆ antiseptic spray
- ◆ ointments for burns and cuts
- ◆ latex gloves

- Other items you may want:

  - ◆ laxative
  - ◆ antidiarrhea medication
  - ◆ activated charcoal (used if advised by the Poison Control Center)
  - ◆ syrup of ipecac (used to induce vomiting if advised by the Poison Control Center)
  - ◆ sunscreen
  - ◆ bug repellent
  - ◆ medicine dropper

- Possible additional medical items:

  - ◆ insulin
  - ◆ allergy medication, including epinephrine for insect allergies
  - ◆ denture needs
  - ◆ contact lenses and supplies
  - ◆ extra eye glasses
  - ◆ heart and high blood pressure medication

## THE VITAL IMPORTANCE OF WATER

Having an adequate water supply during an emergency is a top priority.

- Store water in plastic containers, such as clean soft-drink plastic bottles. Store in a dark place and refill with fresh water every 6 months. Avoid breakable bottles.

- Keep at least a three-day supply of water, or a minimum of three gallons per person.
- If you're at home at the time of the emergency, you may have time to fill tubs and containers with water. This will be very important.
- To improve the taste of stored or boiled water, put the oxygen back into the water by pouring the water back and forth between two containers. (A funnel will be handy.)
- If water needs to be treated before drinking:

  ◆ If you have power, boiling is the safest method. The Federal Emergency Management Agency (FEMA) and the American Red Cross recommend bringing water to a rolling boil for ten minutes. After boiling, the water should be strained through a coffee filter or cheesecloth. Add 16 drops of unscented chlorine bleach to each gallon of water. Let stand for one-half hour. Drinkable water will look clear and smell slightly of chlorine. (The Centers for Disease Control notes that the chlorine treatment alone will kill bacteria but not parasites.)

- Melt ice cubes or use water from undamaged hot water tanks, toilet tanks (not the bowl), and water pipes if you need additional water.

## FOOD

While it is unlikely that you would need it, many experts recommend that you stockpile two weeks' worth of food. The easiest way to do this is to simply buy a little more of what you have on hand anyway.

- For buying "extra," select food that requires no refrigeration, preparation, or cooking, and little or no water. For example, stock up on salt-free crackers, whole-grain cereals, and canned food with high liquid content. Rotate these foods as part of your regular supply so that even in an emergency the food will be as fresh as possible.

- If your electricity goes off, it may be important to conserve your food. The order in which you consume each item will make a difference in how long your supplies last. The first foods you should eat are the perishable foods, including those in your refrigerator that will go bad; then consider eating those in the freezer, though if they've been thawed for any period of time, toss what might have spoiled. Finally the nonperishable foods and staples should be consumed.
- Establish a separate stash of food in case of evacuation. See the following suggestions on what to take with you.

## IN CASE OF EVACUATION:

In the event of an evacuation, you should grab your "Basics" duffel in addition to a larger duffel that should be packed with the following:

- Water to take with you. To have a basic supply, you will want three gallons of water per person. If you live in a hot climate or one of you is nursing or ill, you'll need more water. Have it packed and ready to go in case there is no time to gather water before leaving home.
- Basic bleach for cleaning and for treating water (16 drops per gallon) and a supply of cheesecloth or coffee filters for straining it
- A three-day supply of nonperishable food. High-energy goods such as peanut butter, crackers, granola bars, and trail mix are a good idea. Also shop for:

  - dried foods
  - prepackaged beverages in foil packets or foil-lined boxes

are suitable because they are well sealed and will keep
for a long time
   - powdered or evaporated milk
   - canned meats, fish, fruits, vegetables, and soups
   - instant coffee, tea, and cocoa
   - snack-sized canned goods. These generally have pull-top
     lids, making them handy in an emergency.

- Kitchen accessories:

   - a manual can opener
   - mess kits
   - paper cups
   - plastic utensils
   - utility knife
   - can of cooking fuel if food must be cooked
   - aluminum foil
   - plastic resealable bags

- One complete change of clothing for each member of the
  family, including:

   - sturdy shoes or work boots
   - rain gear
   - hat and gloves
   - sunglasses
   - thermal underwear

- Sanitation and hygiene items

   - toilet paper and paper towels
   - soap, hand sanitizer
   - lip balm
   - shampoo and deodorant
   - toothpaste and toothbrush
   - comb and brush

- Tools and accessories

  - paper and pencil
  - needles and thread
  - pliers
  - duct tape

- Entertainment items

  - games, books, etc.

- Blanket or sleeping bag for each family member

*A special warning from the American Red Cross:* If your power is out, use battery-powered lighting at all times. Don't use candles. According to the Red Cross, accidents with candles frequently compound the disaster by causing fires.

## VERY IMPORTANT

- Take time now to read the instructions and learn to use what you carry in your supplies kit. For example, if you need an EpiPen because someone in the family is allergic, read about what to do with it. Once the emergency occurs, there may be no time to learn.

## EMERGENCY SUPPLIES FOR A PET

- Place the following in an easy-to-carry bag, and keep this bag with your Evacuation Kit:

  - Medications and medical records (including proof of rabies vaccination) in a waterproof container
  - Sturdy leashes or harnesses

- ◆ Food, potable water, bowls, cat litter/pan, and can opener if needed
- ◆ Information on feeding schedules, medical conditions, behavior problems, and the name and number of your veterinarian in case you have to leave your pet in the care of someone else
- ◆ Current photos of your pets in case they get lost.

- Plan how you will travel with your pet. Do you need a crate or a box? If so, you'll want to make a note of that with your disaster supplies.

# Chapter 5

# Insuring Against Disaster

Not a week goes by when the nightly news doesn't carry some report of a disaster. The video clips frequently show a family standing in front of a home that has been gutted by fire or the contents ruined by floodwaters. Sometimes the people are picking through the debris of what used to be their home—finding a framed photo here and a miraculously still intact vase there, wondering how they will ever rebuild after the devastation wrought on their family by the latest earthquake, tornado, or hurricane.

While it takes years to mend the psychological scars any major disaster leaves, the one hope we might have for any family facing catastrophe is that they had adequate insurance coverage and that a check will soon arrive from the insurance company that will give the family the financial backing they will need to start rebuilding their home.

Arranging for insurance coverage is an easy and an important step for you to take so that you and your family aren't caught in an emergency or natural disaster without adequate coverage. When it comes to insuring against disaster, "adequate" is the key word. While many Americans go to bed thinking they are insured, they often wake up to face a flood, a tornado, or a hurricane, and learn that they don't have the coverage needed to protect them against loss or damage to their home and its contents. It pays to be well-informed on this topic.

Whether you own your home or rent a house or apartment, here's what you need to know about buying insurance that will see you through a particularly bad time.

## REEXAMINE YOUR POLICY

Begin by reading your policy, keeping in mind some of the topics in this book. Are you covered for the types of peril that might occur in your area?

If you have a standard homeowners policy, most insurance companies will protect you against fire or lightning; windstorm or hail; explosion; riot or civil commotion; aircraft; vehicles; smoke; vandalism or malicious mischief; theft; damage by glass or safety glazing that is part of a building; volcanic eruption. Some policies also cover damage caused by falling objects, heavy ice, snow, or sleet; three categories of water-related damage from home utilities or appliances; and electrical surge damage. Renters should have personal property coverage for most of the above perils.

People frequently overlook the fact that a basic policy doesn't cover damage from floods, yet floods cause about $2 billion in property damage each year. What's more, a third of all flood claims come from areas that are not prone to floods, where homeowners are unlikely to have thought flood insurance would be necessary.

Flood insurance is available through the National Flood Insurance Program, if you live in a community that has followed federal flood management guidelines. Call your insurance agent to see if you should have this additional coverage. You can buy it locally, or call the program directly (1-888-225-5336) to get the name of agents in your area who will sell it to you. If you live in a participating community, you can buy up to $250,000 coverage for a residence, $500,000 for a commercial building. The average flood policy premium is about $300 for approximately $98,000 of coverage. Don't wait for it to start raining before you buy it; there is a 30-day waiting period before it becomes effective.

Whether you rent or own your home, be sure to ask your agent about contents coverage. It is not automatically included with building coverage.

Also check your auto insurance. You should be covered for damage incurred in a storm, a fire, or a flood.

Earthquake insurance must also be purchased separately. In California, it is available through the state and can be quite costly, but anyone who has ever experienced an earthquake knows that the coverage is a necessity, not an option.

If you have any questions about what is covered, ask your agent to clarify the terms for you.

## BE CERTAIN WHAT YOU'RE GETTING FOR YOUR MONEY

When you buy a household policy, the agent should explain to you what type of coverage you're getting for your money. You also need to evaluate whether or not the amount for which you're covered is still adequate. You may have made household changes since the time you originally purchased the policy.

While it is virtually impossible to emerge from these experiences without some additional out-of-pocket costs, what you want in a good insurance policy is guaranteed replacement coverage—what would it cost to rebuild the house today? Talk to your insurance agent. Each company has a different way of defining guaranteed replacement coverage. Some pay for the full replacement cost of the home no matter what it costs; other insurers set limits, so be sure to ask if you don't remember how your policy works. If you're not happy with the type of arrangement you have, now is the time to change it even if it means switching to another insurance agent.

While most insurance companies will send out an appraiser to estimate the value of your home, you can get a ballpark estimate of the cost of rebuilding by doing a little math: Calculate the square footage of your home and multiply it by local building costs per square foot, a figure you can get over the telephone from your insurance agent. That will give you a general idea of the level of insurance necessary to adequately insure your home.

Take time now to be sure you fully understand the provisions of the policy and that everything that should be insured is adequately covered. You don't want to have to worry about this once you're in the midst of a major storm or other natural disaster.

## PROVIDING PROOF OF WHAT YOU HAVE

While the insurance company will have a general idea of the value of your possessions, you can increase the chance of getting the coverage you deserve by doing a little homework:

- If you have anything of extraordinary value (artwork, jewelry, furs, collectibles), make certain your insurance agent knows about it. Have the items appraised; you may want to purchase a rider to cover them separately. Without a separate rider, a costly diamond necklace is just a nice necklace if it's lost or stolen.
- The next step is to prepare a home inventory. This will help in obtaining insurance settlements and/or tax deductions for losses.

  Why take an inventory? Because you may think you'll remember everything, but you can't. What's more, a detailed record complete with serial numbers will greatly strengthen your opportunity to get as much reimbursement as you can.

  If you still don't think an inventory is necessary, try this test. Sit in your kitchen and make a list of everything you can remember of the furnishings, artwork, and family memorabilia you have in your living room. Now check on how many items you missed.

No one really expects to lose furniture or other belongings in a fire, a burglary, or a tornado, but such events do occur. If disaster struck your home, would you be able to report exactly what you lost to police, to the IRS, or to your insurance company?

- List items, with descriptions, and take pictures or even make a videotape. Make three copies of the documentation. Keep one at home so you can check when it needs to be updated; put one in your safe deposit box; and send one to a relative in another part of the country.
- If you have any questions as you prepare the inventory, call your insurance agent. Remember, the more thorough your inventory, the more valuable it will be in case of a loss.
- To back up your written inventory, photograph each wall of each room with closet or cabinet doors open. On the back of each picture, write the date, the general location, and contents shown.
- In preparing an inventory, use the following form. Just reading the list will make you realize how detailed you need to be.

## INVENTORY RECORD

*For each of the following, list the article, a description of it, the price, and the purchase date.*

### LIVING ROOM

Carpet/rugs _____

_____

Curtains/drapes _____

_____

Sofas _____

_____

Chairs _____

_____

Coffee tables _____

End tables or tables _____

Desk _____

Mirrors, pictures, and wall hangings _____

_____

_____

_____

Clocks _____

Lamps _____

_____

_____

Television/VCR, radio/CD player _____

_____

Records/tapes _____

_____

Books _____

_____

Musical instruments _____

Plants/planters _____

Accessories _____

Other _____

_____

Total _____

## DINING ROOM

Carpet/rugs _____

_____

Curtains/drapes _____

_____

Buffet _____
Tables _____
Chairs _____
China cabinet _____
Silverware _____
Glassware _____
Clock _____
Lamps/fixtures _____
Wall hangings _____

_____

_____

Serving table/cart _____
Other _____

_____

Total _____

## BATHROOM

Clothes hamper _____
Curtains _____
Dressing table _____
Electrical appliances _____

_____

Scale _____
Shower curtains _____
Linens _____
Other _____

_____

Total _____

## KITCHEN

Tables _____

Chairs _____

Curtains _____

Cabinets _____

_____

Lighting fixtures _____

Pots/pans _____

_____

Cutlery & utensils _____

Dishes _____

_____

Appliances (refrigerator, stove, dishwasher, compactor, disposal, etc.) _____

_____

_____

_____

_____

_____

_____

Washer and dryer _____

Small appliances _____

_____

Clocks and radios _____

Other _____

_____

                                        Total _____

## BEDROOMS

Carpet/rugs _____

_____

Curtains/drapes _____

_____

Bookcases _____

_____

Chairs _____

_____

Beds/mattresses/bedding _____

_____

Desk _____

Chests/ dressers/dressing tables _____

_____

_____

_____

Night tables _____

Lamps _____

Pictures/mirrors/wall hangings _____

_____

Clocks/radios/television/CD player _____

_____

_____

Sewing machine _____

Toilet articles _____

Clothing _____

_____

_____

_____

_____

Other _____

_____

_____

Total _____

## GARAGE/BASEMENT/ATTIC

Furniture _____

_____

_____

Luggage/trunks _____

_____

_____

Sports equipment _____

_____

Toys _____

_____

Outdoor games _____

_____

Ornamental lawn items _____

_____

Shovels _____
Spreaders _____
Sprinklers/hoses _____
Lawn mower/wheelbarrow/snowblower _____

_____

_____

Garden tools/supplies _____

_____

_____

Ladders/step stools _____
Workbench _____
Carpentry tools/supplies _____

_____

_____

Canned goods/supplies _____

_____

Pet supplies _____
Other _____

_____

                                        Total _____

## PORCH/PATIO

Chairs _____

_____

Tables _____

_____

Umbrella _____

Floor covering _____
Lamps _____
Outdoor cooking equipment _____
Plants/planters _____
Other _____

_____
Total _____

## WHAT HAPPENS AFTER A DISASTER

If there's been damage to your home, it's up to you to notify the insurance company. An adjuster will be sent to assess the necessary repairs so that payment can be made.

If, however, your community has been devastated by a storm or another natural disaster, companies will generally send out an emergency response team to begin to assess the destruction. (Once you are safe, call your agent or your carrier's 800-number anyway. There's no sense in waiting for them to look for you.) If the President declares the area a disaster, the federal government may also send staffers to help with the workload.

Even if an adjuster appears on the scene quickly, it can still take time to get a check for the full amount of your losses. However, most companies will be prepared to start paying out some money for living expenses.

Your next job will involve getting estimates so that a figure for settlement can be reached. If you're in the midst of a community-wide disaster, the more easily available contractors may not be the most reputable. Ideally, call a contractor you know or one recommended by friends in order to get an accurate and reliable estimate.

Once the adjuster's report is in, the insurance company will give you the amount they are willing to pay. If you feel it's an unfair figure based on the estimates you received, ask for more. There may be some room for negotiation if you have written estimates that explain why a contractor expects the job to cost more.

## BE SURE TO . . .

- Purchase guaranteed replacement coverage for your home and its contents.
- If you experience a fire or community disaster, contact your agent or call the carrier's 800-number as soon as you are safe.
- Request living expenses if you can't stay at home.
- Get your own estimates for the work that needs to be done so that you'll know whether or not the insurance settlement is adequate. You're unlikely to be totally repaid for what it's going to cost you to rebuild, but the closer you can get, the better.

# PART TWO

# SAFETY SPECIFICS

# Chapter 6

# Home Dangers

## Introduction

Home is our oasis, the place where we want to feel safe and far away from the worries of everyday life. Yet 28 percent of fatal accidents occur in the home, and large numbers of people become ill from the hidden dangers within household walls.

Recent news headlines have also made us well aware of the importance of our water supply—whether we're having a drink of water at a county fair or turning on the tap in our own home. How can we be sure the water we drink is safe? And what can we do if it isn't?

Another section in this chapter addresses garbage. Although it's been a long time since ecology became a priority on political agendas, after reading about what we're doing to our world, you may begin to feel that we're not adequately safeguarding our environment. People used to worry about living next to Superfund sites with toxic waste. Now simply having a town landfill presents certain dangers.

A final section talks about what to do if you wake up one morning and nothing works—a systems breakdown on a household or community-wide scale.

This chapter of the book will tell you what you can do to make your home environment safer, and it provides solutions when something goes wrong. Some of these solutions involve working with neighbors and prodding the government. To keep our children (and our children's children) truly safe, we all need to work together, with long-term goals in mind.

# Fire Safety

Fire. Destructive, devastating, and dangerous, yet almost all of us tend to be cavalier about it, forgetting to check our smoke alarms regularly, or sitting through a blaring fire alarm at the office because we assume the warning is false.

Then we see an evening news story about a major fire in an office building, or we hear the reporter talk of a home that was totally gutted because a family member tried to fight the fire himself instead of calling 9-1-1. At these times, our certainty that "it couldn't happen to me" fades, and we wonder—"Could it?"

If you're serious about safety, you need to address fire safety in two ways. First, make certain your environment is at low risk for fire by checking your wiring and taking other electrical fire safety measures; and second, create an emergency plan (including a no-fail habit of checking out any alarms that sound) that will allow you and your family to escape a fire in time.

## ELECTRICAL SAFETY

Approximately 500 people lose their lives each year by electrocution in or around the home. In addition, there are approximately 190,000 fires of electrical origin, resulting in about 1,000 deaths and 11,000 injuries each year, not to mention massive property destruction. These are sobering statistics, particularly in light of the fact that electrical problems are almost totally preventable.

- If you're living in an older home or one that may have been partially wired by a previous owner (not necessarily an electrician), schedule a visit from an electrical contractor. Ask him to:

  ◆ Check that your wiring is done to code; even one jerry-rigged set of wires done by a home handyman can be enough to set fire to your entire home.

  ◆ Ask if the electrical capacity is adequate for today's wired world. Particularly with the increasing use of computers and the ever-growing number of electrical products we're bringing into our homes, there is every reason to think that most families would be wise to upgrade their circuitry. Trying to use more appliances than the system can handle is hazardous. A television picture that "shrinks," fuses that blow, or circuits that trip are indications that this should be a household priority.

  ◆ If a switch or an outlet seems warm, unplug everything connected to it and have it checked. This may be a sign of bad wiring.

  ◆ Make certain that your circuit breakers (or fuses) are labeled as to what they control. The electrician can help you.

- If Ground Fault Circuit Interrupters (GFCI) outlets aren't currently in place in your bathrooms or kitchen, have them put in. If there is a sudden change in the amount of electricity flowing into an outlet (as would happen if a hair dryer or other appliance were to be dropped into water), then the GFCI immediately cuts current to the outlet, greatly reducing the risk of electrocution.

- Electrical wiring is one home project that should be left to a licensed professional. Though you may have a general idea of what to do, the results can be disastrous if you make an error.

- Make a survey of your home, checking lamps and appliances:

  - ◆ Use only appliances that bear the Underwriters Laboratory (UL) seal.
  - ◆ Use safety caps on all unused outlets and safety covers on all used ones if you have young children.
  - ◆ Don't knot appliance cords.
  - ◆ If you need an electrical cord tacked out of the way, ask a professional to do it for you. He'll have the type of stapler that can fit around the wire without cutting into it. Using a household staple gun or a nail to tack the wire may result in your cutting through the cord, creating a fire hazard.
  - ◆ Don't run any cords (computer cords, extension cords, etc.) across traffic ways or under carpets. The traffic over a hidden cord or the weight of a piece of furniture can damage the cord, which can lead to heat or a spark and a fire. If you need a lamp on a sofa table that "floats" in the middle of the room, spend the money to have an electrician put an outlet in the floor.
  - ◆ Extension cords should be used only temporarily and with care. Approximately 600 mouth-burn injuries occur each year to children who bite or teethe on an extension cord.
  - ◆ Avoid the use of multi-plug or "octopus" adapters (devices that allow you to plug additional electrical equipment into a socket). It is dangerous for a single outlet to carry a heavier electrical load than that for which it is wired. Get an electrician to add an extra outlet.

- The dangers of halogen torchère lights (tall floor lamps that use high-wattage halogen bulbs) became known to the public when jazz great Lionel Hampton's Manhattan apartment was set on fire in 1997, and the cause was a halogen lamp that ignited a piece of clothing. While these lamps are now more closely regulated than they were before, it's worth paying attention to how you use them—they do burn much hotter than an incandescent bulb. A 300-watt halogen can burn as hot as 970°F while a 150-watt incandescent reaches only about 340°.

- Here are some ways to use any type of lamp safely:

  - ◆ Place the lamp where it can't be tipped over by children, pets, or a strong draft. Avoid placing it by open windows where drapery can be blown onto the bulb.
  - ◆ Never use a bulb of a different type or higher wattage than is indicated in the manufacturer's instructions.
  - ◆ Wait until the bulb cools before trying to replace it.
  - ◆ Avoid leaving lamps of 100 watts or more on when you leave the room or aren't at home.
  - ◆ Never drape anything over a lamp.
  - ◆ Lamps with a dimmer switch should be set lower than the maximum capacity whenever possible.
  - ◆ Keep lamps away from bunk beds or bed canopies where bedding may get too close to the bulb.

- The holidays are one of the most dangerous times of year. Before plugging in that old string of lights, consider their condition and whether or not the plug can carry the load. Turn holiday lights off when you're not going to be home or after you've gone to bed.
- Add the local power company's telephone number to your list of emergency numbers.

## ELECTRICAL FIRST AID

If someone gets hurt in an electrical accident, they may still be holding the item that caused the shock. Don't touch the person, or you may become part of the circuit. Use something dry and nonmetal such as a wooden broom handle to push or pull the victim away from the power source. Once you have freed the person from the contact, call 9-1-1 and begin normal first aid procedures.

## GENERAL FIRE SAFETY

Fire is the first cause of death at home for children under the age of 15, and roughly 80 percent of all fire deaths occur when people are asleep. For that reason, it's very important to take precautions so that your home is as safe as possible.

- There's nothing safe about anything that involves an open flame. Be extremely careful with candles:

  - Never leave them unattended.
  - Don't place them where anything can blow across the flame.
  - Place them in a holder where the candles won't tip, and where, if the hot wax drips, it won't burn anyone or anything.

- Be very careful with cigarettes:

  - No one should smoke in bed.
  - Provide deep ashtrays for smokers.
  - If someone has been smoking in your house, check under the couch and chair cushions for smoldering cigarettes before you go to bed.

- Fireplaces are a warm and wonderful addition to any household, but be respectful of your responsibility once a fire is lit:

  - Keep combustibles away from the fire.
  - Use a firescreen correctly.
  - Never go to bed before the fire is fully extinguished.

- Keep portable heaters at least three feet away from combustibles: paper, bedding, clothes, or curtains. Always turn the heater off when you go to sleep or leave the house.
- Make certain the television has open space around it to prevent overheating.
- Don't ever leave anything on the stove burner unattended.
- Store gasoline and other flammables outside in tight, labeled metal containers. Don't store them inside your home or basement. If a fire should start, the flammable material will increase the speed and danger of the fire.
- Keep matches out of the hands of unsupervised children. Over time teach them match safety:

  - Introduce children to the concept that a match is a tool, not a toy. Talk to them about the appropriate use of fire.
  - When your child is old enough (has good motor skills and the desire to learn), teach him the correct way to light a match—by closing the cover of the matchbook or matchbox. Emphasize the importance of striking away from the body. Also teach the importance of properly discarding a match. By teaching children the proper use of matches, you lessen the chance that they will be harmed by trying to teach themselves how to use them.

## AVOID BURNS

- Keep your hot water heater set below 120°F.
- For young children, always check the temperature of the bathwater.
- Be careful when removing a cover from anything that's been in the microwave. The vapors released can be extremely hot.
- Cook with pot handles turned in so that someone walking past the stove won't brush against a handle and knock the pot off the stove.

- Cook only in tight sleeves.
- Don't store things above or behind the stove. People sometimes get burned when they are reaching across hot burners.

## SMOKE ALARMS AND FIRE EXTINGUISHERS

- Place smoke detectors on each floor of the house and within 15 feet of sleeping areas. If family members sleep with their doors closed, then a smoke alarm belongs inside the bedroom.
- A detector outside the kitchen with a three-minute delay will provide enough time for you to air the room out if you burn the vegetables.
- Use the test button to test your smoke alarms once a month.
- If your smoke alarms aren't hard-wired into an alarm system, be sure to change the batteries annually.
- Replace any type of smoke alarm every ten years.
- Keep a 12–18 inch "A-B-C" fire extinguisher in the kitchen. It is appropriate for small grease, electrical, or waste paper fires. (Baking soda is also good on grease fires.) Before trying to fight a fire yourself—even a small one—call 9-1-1 first. A fire can get out of hand quickly. If you should succeed in putting it out yourself, the fire department will be on hand to be certain it's totally out.

## CREATE A FAMILY ESCAPE PLAN

- Draw a floor plan of your home. Walk through your home or apartment with family members, noting how you would exit no matter where you were. In some rooms you may be able to get out a door and a window, and some rooms may actually have more than one door for getting out of the space quickly.

- Consider escape ladders for sleeping areas on the second and third floors. Learn how to use them.
- If you have window guards on your windows, consider how they open. If you need a key, find a nearby place to store it so that it will be accessible in an emergency.
- Select a safe meeting place outside the home if your family has to escape from a fire. The home of a nearby neighbor is ideal because that provides you with phone access.
- Conduct a home fire drill at least twice a year. It's best to do it at night as well as during the day, and practice different routes as you exit the house.

## RESPOND TO ANY AND ALL ALARMS

If you hear a fire alarm, you need to respond immediately. While you don't necessarily need to dash for the fire stairs instantly, you do need to track down whether or not there is a real emergency.

- In a public building or a hotel, where you may not be able to locate anyone very quickly, don't take a chance—get out.
- At work, know how to reach or find the maintenance staff so that you can check with them quickly. You may find that the system is being tested or that there is construction in the building but that everything is under control, or you may learn you'd better head for an exit. (Have the maintenance number at your fingertips; if you have to call through a building operator, you may find the operator's system is tied up with other people who are asking similar questions.)
- At home, start looking for the source of the trouble. While both water and dust can cause a smoke alarm to malfunction,

you need to locate the smoke alarm that has gone off, and determine what's gone wrong. A 3:00 A.M. trek to all the smoke alarms in a house isn't fun, but it is necessary to safeguard your family.

- Teach children to respond *whenever they hear an alarm*, no matter what their friends are doing. Again, the proper response is to find out what is happening, not necessarily to make an immediate dash for the street. (While teachers tend to be excellent at managing alarms—false and otherwise—sometimes after-school activity personnel can become blasé about false alarms. It's still appropriate for a student to suggest that someone needs to be sure it's really false.)

## IN CASE OF FIRE

- As soon as you spot fire, call "Fire!" and get family members out of the house immediately. Even if the fire is a small one confined to a single room at the time you notice it, everyone needs to leave right away. Homes and lives have been lost when people stay to try to put out the fire themselves and neglect to place priority on "life over property." Once out of the house, call 9-1-1. Don't stay inside to make the phone call.
- Crawl low if it's smoky.
- If you must open a closed door on your way, feel the door first. Use the more sensitive back of your hand to feel for temperature. If it's warm, you may want to go another way. If you must stay put, open a window for ventilation and put something in the window so that firefighters will see you. If there is a phone in the room, telephone to let them know your whereabouts.

## IF YOU CATCH ON FIRE

*Don't panic, and don't run.* Running will only increase the flames. Instead . . .

- Stop! Drop! Roll! Continue to roll until you have completely put out the fire.
- Remove clothing from any burned area, but don't pull away cloth that sticks.
- Flush any burned area with cold water. Quick cooling may prevent a severe burn.
- Don't apply grease or ointments.
- Cover with a sterile pad or a clean sheet.
- Seek medical attention.

## HIGH-RISE FIRE

Even when you're simply arriving for an appointment at a high-rise office building or checking into a hotel, note the fire exits. Mentally map out two escape routes.

When selecting a hotel, ask if the building has a sprinkler system to deal with fires; fire safety experts often request a room no higher than the seventh floor because exit is easier (by ladder or by stairs) from the lower floors. Once you've been assigned a room, count the doors between your room and the fire exits in case you have to escape in the dark.

Once the alarm sounds, you need to decide what your options are:

- If the path seems clear for leaving the room, go to the stairwell (which should be smoke-free). Don't ever get into an elevator. Don't walk upright. Heat and smoke rise, and the passageway may be smoky enough to harm you.
- If the room is full of smoke, crawl on your hands and knees.

The best air and visibility are found 12–24 inches off the floor. If possible, put a wet handkerchief over your mouth and nose as an improvised filter.

- If your door is hot, call the operator or the emergency number and tell them where you are. If the phones aren't working, use a flashlight or hang a light-colored towel or sheet out the window to signal for help. Fill the bathtub with water; it will be useful for dousing towels or flaming clothing. Seal door cracks and vents with wet towels, and shut off fans and air conditioners.

- *If you are in a "fireproof" high-rise, the advice changes:*

    ◆ If the fire is in your apartment, leave and *close the door behind you*.
    ◆ If the fire is elsewhere in the building, resist the urge to flee down the stairwell. Stay in your apartment. The fire department will come and get you. Use the phone to call and say where you are, or put something in the window. In a New York City tragedy, several people died in a stairwell 8–10 floors above the affected apartment, while trying to make their way downstairs. The unit where the fire started was damaged, but because the apartment door was left open, smoke spread to the fire stairs. The apartments on either side of the unit where the fire started weren't damaged at all.

- If smoke is coming in from outside, turn off the air conditioner and close the windows.

- When you call 9-1-1, give your name and address and the location of your apartment (floor number as well as direction: "South side of the building," for example).

## THREE TOP TIPS TO TEACH CHILDREN ABOUT FIRE SAFETY

1. Have children practice "Stop, Drop, Roll" regularly. Practice with them.
2. Teach your children to unplug electrical items safely, holding on to the plug itself, not tugging on the cord.
3. Teach children that fire is extremely dangerous. If an alarm sounds, they **must** respond to it.

## HOT BUTTON

- Install smoke alarms in your house, and buy fire extinguishers as well.
- Do a house check for fire hazards and electrical problems.
- Practice fire drills with the family.

# Preventing Accidental Poisonings and Falls

Accidental poisonings and falls are the two top hazards in the home. Approximately 40 children between ages of one and five die each year from accidental poisonings, and Poison Control Centers nationwide receive nearly 2 million calls each year. Older adults are subject to falls, and they are the number one disabling accident in the home. On both counts, it's worth paying attention to what you can do to make your home safer.

## PREVENTING HOUSEHOLD POISONINGS

Children learn about the world by exploring, and unfortunately, many of the things they find they put in their mouths. For that reason, it's vital that you take every precaution to safeguard your children.

Substances that present a particular danger to children include medications (everything from vitamins to sleeping pills to prescription medicines), corrosive chemicals (cleansers, detergents, drain openers, etc.), toiletries (nail polish removers or mouthwash), and pesticides.

Here are some room-by-room safety tips:

### In the Kitchen:

- Post your local Poison Control Center number.
- Be sure you have Syrup of Ipecac and activated charcoal on hand in case you should need either one. (Don't ever give either of these unless instructed to do so by the PCC. Administering the wrong one can be very dangerous.)
- Make certain that all harmful products are in child-resistant caps and in their original packaging. If your child should ingest something, most bottles of hazardous materials say what the antidote is.
- Keep any type of hazardous substance up high or in a cabinet or drawer with a safety latch. Some children are so precocious that they can get through to almost anything. If you have one of these kids, then you'll have to consider a safety latch on a high cabinet. It's inconvenient, but not as inconvenient as a trip to the emergency room.
- Don't ever store pesticides or chemicals near food.

### In the Bathroom:

- All medicines should have child-resistant closures.
- Toss all out-of-date prescriptions. They can be dangerous for both children and adults.
- Keep all medicines in their original containers with their original labels.
- Only give medication to the person for whom it is prescribed. Don't trade among family members.

### In the Basement or Garage:

- Store pesticides and chemicals in locked cabinets, preferably in an out-of-the-way area of the house such as the garage or basement. In a survey conducted by the Environmental Protection Agency, it was revealed that 47 percent of all households with children under the age of five had at least one pesticide stored in an unlocked cabinet within the reach of children.
- Always store poisons in their original packages so it's clear to you, the child, and any other caregiver that a poison is in the container.
- Before applying pesticides to the yard or any household plants, get children and their toys away from the area and follow the directions carefully.

## WHEN TO CALL THE POISON CONTROL CENTER

Almost 70 percent of the poisonings that occur can be handled at home if you call the PCC right away. However, if the poisoning is more serious, then it's vital that you act immediately. Delaying treatment only increases the risk.

- Call the PCC under the following circumstances:

  - When you think your child has been exposed to a poison.
  - If your child seems abnormally drowsy or sluggish.
  - You notice mysterious stains or burns around his mouth.
  - You smell something strange on your child's breath.
  - You catch your child playing with a bottle of medicine or a dangerous household product.
  - *Call immediately to get instructions.*

- If the poison is on the skin or in the eye, start flushing the area with running water for 15–20 minutes while waiting for help or additional instructions.

## ONE VITAL WARNING

While you're locking up those poisons, give some thought to any guns you might have in the home. Keep them unloaded, and lock them up.

## PREVENTING FALLS

Falls are the biggest cause of household accidents resulting in disability. While the young and the elderly are more prone to falling, accidents can happen to anyone. Here's what you can do:

### *General Safety*

- Secure area rugs, especially those on wood, ceramic tile, or linoleum floors. Secure them with a piece of foam carpet backing, double-sided tape, or a rubber pad available at many carpet and department stores. Check all area rugs to make certain none have turned-up corners or anything else that might present a hazard.
- Use night-lights everywhere anyone might wander during the night. Lack of visibility is a major cause of falls.
- Check your home for electrical cords or anything that might cause someone to trip.
- To prevent little ones from falling from windows, get window guards for all windows above the first floor, and don't let children lean on screens.
- Always strap babies and toddlers into their highchairs and strollers, and don't ever leave them in a high place unattended.

### *Stairs and Halls:*

- Use safety gates if you have babies or toddlers.
- Keep toys and other items off stairs and out of hallways.
- Make sure you have handrails on all staircases, including outdoor steps to and from porches.
- Keep the stairs clear.

### In the Bathroom:

- Nonslip bath mats should be inside and outside the tub and shower.
- Install grab bars for getting out of the tub. These are helpful for people at any age.

## HOT BUTTON

- Keeping children safe from poisons involves proper and safe storage as well as careful supervision.
- Homes can be made safer in order to prevent falls. After surveying your home for dangers, make adjustments right away.

# Chemical Emergencies

In Weyauwega, Wisconsin, the derailment of a freight train and the toppling of fourteen tanker cars carrying liquid propane fuel set off a massive explosion and fire and led to the complete evacuation of the community. This type of chemical accident could happen almost anywhere. More than 278,000 plants and facilities in the United States generate, transport, treat, store, or dispose of hazardous chemicals such as chlorine, propane, and ammonia.

Though the evacuation of a town is very dramatic, equally serious are the types of chemical accidents that happen right in our own home when we spill pesticide on ourselves while gardening, or discover that a child has gotten hold of and may have ingested a household cleanser.

Here's what you need to know to safeguard your family.

## ABOUT HAZARDOUS SUBSTANCES

Hazardous materials are chemical substances that if released or misused can pose a threat to the environment. These chemicals are used in industry, agriculture, medicine, research, and in our own homes. They range from commercial pesticides and industrial explosives to spray cleaners and nail polish remover.

Even without seeing or smelling anything unusual, you can be exposed to chemicals. There are three means of exposure:

- breathing the chemical
- swallowing contaminated food, water, or medication
- touching the chemical, or coming into contact with clothing or items that have touched the chemical.

The most common chemical accidents occur in our own homes, and they can be prevented. (Also refer to "Home Safety: Accidental Falls and Poisonings" for additional information.)

## PREVENTING HOME EMERGENCIES AND PROTECTING THE ENVIRONMENT

- The best way to avoid chemical accidents is to read and follow the directions for use, storage, and disposal of the product. Mixing products can be hazardous.
- Keep all medicines, cosmetics, cleaning products, and other chemicals out of sight and out of reach of children. Small children consuming medicines is the most common chemical emergency.
- Flush old medicines or those not being used down the toilet.
- Store household chemicals according to instructions.
- Avoid mixing common household products. Some, such as ammonia and bleach, can create toxic gases.

- Always read the directions before using; and read instructions about disposal.
- To avoid inhaling dangerous vapors, don't use chemicals in a confined space. Work in an area where you can open the windows.
- How we dispose of home chemicals can have a direct result on our local water supply or the environment. If you have any questions about how to dispose of products, contact the company.

  - Small amounts of the following products can be safely poured down the drain with plenty of water: antifreeze, bathroom and glass cleaner, bleach, drain cleaner, household disinfectant, detergent, rubbing alcohol, upholstery cleaner, and toilet bowl cleaner.
  - Small amounts of the following should be disposed of by wrapping the container in newspapers and plastic and placing it in the trash: brake fluid, car wax or polish, dish and laundry soap, drain cleaner, fertilizer, furniture and floor polish, insect repellent, nail polish, oven cleaner, paint thinners and strippers, pesticides, power cleaners, water-based paint, and wood preservatives.
  - Dispose of the following products at a recycling center or collection site: kerosene, motor or fuel oil, car battery or battery acid, diesel fuel transmission fluid, large amounts of paint, paint thinner or stripper, power steering fluid, turpentine, gun cleaning solvents, and tires.
  - Empty spray cans by pressing the button until nothing comes out, then place the can in the trash. Don't place the can in any place where it will be burned; heat will cause it to explode.

- Never smoke near household chemicals, and never use cleaning solutions, hair sprays, etc. around an open flame such as a candle or pilot light.

- If a chemical spills, clean it up carefully, protecting your eyes and skin. Allow the rags to evaporate outdoors, then dispose of them by wrapping in a newspaper inside a plastic bag. Dispose of them with your trash.
- Don't store chemicals. Buy small quantities to reduce the need to store them and dispose of the excess.
- Keep an A-B-C rated fire extinguisher in your home and car, and get training from your fire department on how to use this model.
- Post the Poison Control Center telephone number on all telephones.

## CHEMICAL POISONING

If someone has ingested or been exposed to a chemical, they may exhibit some of the following symptoms: difficulty breathing; irritation of the eyes, skin, throat, or respiratory tract; changes in skin color; headache or blurred vision; dizziness; clumsiness or lack of coordination; cramps or diarrhea.

If you find someone who appears to have been injured from chemical exposure, call 9-1-1, your local emergency number, or the Poison Control Center.

## MANAGING A HOME CHEMICAL EMERGENCY

- If a chemical comes into contact with the eye, take immediate action. Flush the eye with clear, lukewarm water for a minimum of 15 minutes unless authorities instruct you otherwise. Continue the cleansing process even if the victim indicates he or she is no longer feeling any pain. Then seek medical attention. The same process should be followed for chemical burns, bathing the affected skin in cool water for 15–30 minutes. Also contact 9-1-1.

- If there is danger of a fire or explosion, get out of the house immediately. Call the fire department from a neighbor's. Don't risk staying in the house.
- Stay away from the home to avoid the possibility of breathing toxic fumes.
- Wash hands, arms, or other parts of the body that may have been exposed to the chemical. These can be irritating until they are washed off.
- Discard clothing that may have been contaminated.

## WHAT TO DO IN A MAJOR CHEMICAL EMERGENCY

As with any type of major emergency, you need to keep in mind your evacuation plan and know what method your community would use to warn citizens of a major problem in the area.

- If you hear a siren or warning signal, start listening carefully to radio or television for further emergency information.
- Follow instructions carefully. Your own and your family's well-being will depend on it. The authorities will inform you of:

  - the type of health hazard
  - the area affected
  - how to protect yourself
  - evacuation routes (if necessary)
  - shelter locations
  - type and location of medical facilities
  - the phone numbers if you should need extra help

- Only call EMS, 9-1-1 or the operator for life-threatening emergencies. In circumstances such as this, the phone lines frequently become overwhelmed.

## HOW TO SHELTER IN PLACE

In some circumstances, you may be told to "shelter in place." This is an effort to maintain your safety while keeping you at home. If these are the instructions:

- Close all windows and vents and turn off all fans and heating or cooling systems; shut the fireplace damper. Take family members and pets to an aboveground room with the fewest number of windows and doors. (Heavier chemicals may seep into basements even when they are closed off, so don't go to the basement.)
- Listen to radio or television or an NOAA Weather Radio for further instructions.
- Take your "Basics" duffel and your emergency supplies with you.
- While gathering your family, cover your mouth and nose with a damp cloth.
- Immediately after the announcement is issued, fill bathtubs and large containers with water and turn off the intake valve to the house. Water supplies may become contaminated.
- Await further instructions.

## EVACUATION DURING A CHEMICAL EMERGENCY

If you are told to evacuate, take your "Basics" duffel and your evacuation duffel and leave home as directed. Take only the routes specified; a shortcut may expose you to hazardous materials.

- Listen carefully to instructions so that you'll be certain about what areas are evacuating, what routes to travel, and where to go.
- You might be told to leave immediately, or you may have time to pack some essentials. If you are given time, seal

your home from exposure to contaminants. Close windows, shut vents, and close fireplace dampers.

- Check to be certain neighbors can get out as well.
- Take only one vehicle to the evacuation site. Traffic may be heavy and families who take more than one car may prevent others from getting out at all.
- While driving, close car windows and air vents and turn off the heater and air conditioner.

## AFTERWARD

Return home only when authorities say it is safe. Follow instructions concerning the safety of food and water.

Clean up as directed. Local officials will know the composition of the hazardous material and will be able to tell you how to clean up and dispose of it.

## IF YOU ARE AT THE SCENE OF A CHEMICAL ACCIDENT

- Call 9-1-1 to report the location of the accident immediately.
- Move away from the accident scene as soon as possible to minimize your exposure. Help others move away as well.
- Try to avoid inhaling gases, fumes, or smoke. If possible, cover your mouth with a cloth.
- Stay away from the spilled substance and avoid touching it.
- Accident victims should not be touched until the hazardous material has been identified. Do everything you can to make it easy for emergency personnel to get to the victims as soon as possible.
- Chemicals may be carried by air, gravity, or water, so try to stay upstream, uphill, and upwind of the accident.

## TWO TOP TIPS TO TEACH CHILDREN
## ABOUT CHEMICAL HAZARDS

1. While locking up chemicals and medicines is your responsibility, you can also talk to children about the fact that these substances are "yukky."
2. In a major accident, tell them that it's vital that they follow all instructions.

## HOT BUTTON

- Take precautions around your household for the careful storage and disposal of all chemicals.
- Use natural products whenever possible, to avoid having chemicals around the house.
- In a major chemical accident, tune in to radio or television right away, and follow the exact instructions of emergency personnel.

# Carbon Monoxide and Radon

Invisible and deadly, carbon monoxide and radon can occur anywhere. They are potentially harmful, but totally remediable. That's why it's wise to learn about them and take any necessary action now.

## ABOUT CARBON MONOXIDE

Carbon monoxide poisoning causes about 2100 unintentional deaths in the United States each year, and more than 5000 people go to hospital emergency rooms for treatment. Yet many more people are made ill from lower levels of the invisible gas, and they don't even realize why they feel perpetually tired or seem to be suffering flu-like symptoms.

Carbon monoxide is a colorless, odorless, tasteless, deadly gas. While it's an important element in our world because plants need it to survive, it's deadly if you are exposed to too much of it. It inhibits your blood's capacity to carry oxygen throughout the body, actually suffocating your tissues and organs.

Anyone can be sickened by carbon monoxide, but children, pregnant women, the unborn, and the elderly are at the highest risk.

Carbon monoxide can come into the home through a faulty furnace, wood-burning stove, range, water heater, fireplace, or any device that burns combustible fuel. Starting a car in a closed garage that is attached to the house can contribute to the problem as well.

## SYMPTOMS

Symptoms of carbon monoxide poisoning are similar to the flu but are generally more serious, including headache, fatigue, nausea, dizziness, irregular breathing, mental confusion. If no help arrives, the victim will become unconscious and die.

## PREVENTION

- Have your furnace and heating system inspected and serviced annually by a heating, ventilating, and air conditioning (HVAC) company.
- All fuel combustion appliances should be vented directly outdoors.
- Be sure that fresh air circulates in your home through a vent or a window.
- Never run an automobile in the garage or any other type of enclosed space.

- Have your chimney and flue cleaned professionally. Even if you don't use the fireplace regularly, your chimney is carrying out all the exhaust from your furnace; a dangerous buildup can occur in the lining of your chimney if it isn't tended to periodically. A cleaning every other year will take care of most situations, but ask your HVAC expert what he recommends based on your climate and system.
- Make sure the burner flames on your furnace and stove burn blue, not yellow-orange.
- Never use your gas range or oven for heating the room.
- Never use grills or hibachis inside your home.
- Never operate gas-burning appliances in a closed room.

## THE IMPORTANCE OF DETECTORS

Every home needs a carbon monoxide detector. Multilevel homes should have one detector on each level. It's particularly important to have one located near the bedrooms. They should be installed between "outlet level" (about 15 inches from the floor) and six to seven feet high. They should not be installed in garages, kitchens, furnace rooms, or humid areas because in these areas you are more likely to get false alarms.

- Install detectors at least 15 feet away from a furnace or gas appliance, and avoid installing detectors close to a fan, swamp cooler, or other fresh or turbulent air sources, as these elements will prevent the detector from giving an accurate reading.
- Always test your carbon monoxide detectors when you check the smoke detectors.

## WHAT YOU SHOULD KNOW ABOUT RADON

Radon is a naturally occurring radioactive gas that can be emitted from surrounding soil into the home. You can't see it, taste it, or smell it, but if it's present in elevated levels, it poses a health risk. Radon is the second leading cause of lung cancer, after smoking.

As radon breaks down, it forms radioactive decay products. As you breathe, these can become trapped in your lungs and over time can damage lung tissue. Smokers with radon in the house are at particular risk.

The EPA and the Surgeon General have recommended that all residences (except apartments above the second floor) be tested for radon.

To test your home, purchase an EPA-approved kit (available at hardware stores). Short-term testing can take 2–90 days; long-range testing can take 90 days to a year.

If your radon level is high, a good contractor will know what can be done. It generally involves some sealing of the basement, combined with a method for providing better ventilation. If you don't know anyone in your area to consult, call the Environmental Protection Agency office in your area, and they'll have suggestions.

## HOT BUTTON

- Install carbon monoxide detectors without delay. Carbon monoxide is deadly, and you don't want to run the risk of accidental poisoning.
- Have your house tested for radon. If there is a problem, it can be fixed.

# Lead-based Paint

Lead is a toxic substance that is practically unavoidable in today's environment. It is found in water, soil, certain ceramic dishes, and especially in the lead-painted walls, window frames, doors, and moldings of an estimated 57 million homes in the United States.

Once prized as a bonding agent for paint, lead was valued as a paint additive for other reasons as well. For exterior work, it was particularly resistant to damage from sunlight, and it was so toxic that mildew would not grow on it. Indoors it was simply more durable. Lead in paint was a selling point from the early years of this century until 1978, when it was discovered to be hazardous and was banned.

The dust and chips from lead-based paint are dangerous when swallowed or inhaled. The smallest lead dust particles cannot be seen, but they are particularly dangerous to young children and pregnant women.

If you live in a home built before 1978, there is a high probability that there is some lead in your home, possibly in the paint or in the soldered pipe joints.

Because lead paint can flake off every time you open and close a window or open a painted kitchen cabinet, it is certainly a hazard of which you should be aware. If the lead level in your household is low and your children are older, you may decide to wait and deal with the problem when you repaint or remodel. However, if the lead level is high, you'll want to take appropriate measures right away.

The first step is determining whether you have a problem at all.

## CALLING IN A PROFESSIONAL

Only a professional can determine whether you have a lead problem in your house, and if so, on what surfaces.

To find a lead inspector, contact your local health department, or the National Lead Information Center Clearinghouse at (800) 424-LEAD for suggestions on locating a reputable inspection service in your area. (Do-it-yourself kits are available, but government officials question their accuracy.)

Testing for lead formerly involved removing chips of paint from numerous surfaces—sometimes as many as 150—and having them evaluated at a laboratory. This was laborious and expensive (as much as $4000). Now most inspectors will test the surfaces of your home by using a portable X-ray fluorescence (XRF) machine, which measures the amount of lead in the paint. Charges are generally $300–$500.

## IF LEAD IS FOUND

- Consider what surfaces have been identified as having a high content. If doors are the primary culprit, they can be removed and sent out to be stripped. Window sashes can be removed, and a stripping solution can be used to remove the paint.

- If the problem is more pervasive, have the removal or encapsulation done by a lead-abatement service worker who has been trained to protect your family and home from exposure. The person who inspected your home may run such a service or will know of these services. If you want to get other names for price comparison, consult your local health department, or check the Yellow Pages under "lead." When you speak to the lead abatement services, ask for several references. When you call, ask if they have taken an EPA-accredited course on safe and proper procedures for lead removal.

- Have young children take a blood test. According to the EPA, one out of every six preschoolers suffers from lead poisoning. Children under the age of six are most vulnerable. (Refer to "Understanding Lead Levels" at the end of this section for information on the meaning of various lead levels.)

- By law, a professional must take great care in the removal of the lead-based paint, but here are two additional precautions you can take:

  - ◆ While the work is taking place, be sure that all heating and air-conditioning systems are turned off so that the dust is not blown through the home. In addition, keep nonworkers, particularly children and pregnant women, away from the work area.
  - ◆ Though the person you have hired should be responsible for cleaning up, if for any reason you are doing so, the only household detergent effective at cleaning up lead dust is powdered high phosphate automatic dishwasher detergent. Lead-specific cleaning products are also available at some paint and hardware stores.

- After the final cleanup, areas should be tested for lead dust contamination to make certain that the area is now lead-free.

## SYMPTOMS

Lead can affect children's developing nervous systems, causing reduced IQ and learning disabilities. Adults are not as susceptible, but when they do show high lead levels, they may notice symptoms varying from headaches to high blood pressure and a long list of other possible symptoms.

Exposure to lead-based paint is not the only cause for high lead levels in children. Children can also get lead poisoning from such places as water systems that have lead pipes or playgrounds that are located near highways where the pollution level is high. Many experts are pushing for all children under the age of six to be tested every year. Lead poisoning can be treated if it's found early.

## UNDERSTANDING LEAD LEVELS

If your child has slightly elevated levels of lead in the blood, talk to your pediatrician. Recent research seems to indicate that for lead exposure to cause permanent damage, it must occur over an extended period of time. By following the recommendations of your doctor, you should be able to prevent your child from suffering any permanent ill effects.

According to the Centers for Disease Control and Prevention in Atlanta, here's how to respond to elevated lead-level readings:

*10–14 micrograms of lead per deciliter of blood:* No action necessary other than retesting child within a couple of months.

*15–19 micrograms:* Doctors are told to educate parents as to how to clean up household dust, which might contain lead. Parents are also told to encourage children to eat food rich in iron and calcium, which helps prevent the absorption of lead. If elevated levels persist after retesting in a few months, a professional inspector should be called in to identify the source.

*20 micrograms and above:* Begin immediately to identify and eliminate the source of lead in the home by encapsulating it or having it removed.

*45 micrograms and above:* Medical intervention may be necessary. One treatment is chelation, a pharmacological therapy, administered orally or intravenously, that draws lead out of the blood.

## ONE TOP TIP TO TEACH YOUR CHILDREN ABOUT LEAD-BASED PAINT

Try to prevent little ones from picking at paint or eating it, and keep cribs away from window or door frames where there might be flaking paint. Toddler boredom during nap time can lead to ingesting flakes of paint.

HOT BUTTON

- Take the first step by getting your house tested. Then you can decide what to do.

## Your Water Supply

We take for granted the fact that we can turn on the tap water in our own home or go to a public drinking fountain and obtain a refreshing, uncontaminated drink of water. Then something happens to prove otherwise. We need to go back only as far as 1993 when 400,000 people in Milwaukee were sickened from a parasite called cryptosporidium in the public water supply and 100 people died; or to 1999 when well water at a county fair in New York State led to at least 804 cases of illness and several deaths from E. coli.

An informal estimate from the Centers for Disease Control and Prevention indicates that from 200,000 to 1,300,000 Americans are sickened by microbes in drinking water each year, with 50–1200 losing their lives as a result.

And while there are many safeguards in place for public water systems as well as private wells to keep them clean and pollution-free during normal circumstances, there is definitely room for improvement. Here's a little background on where we are when it comes to public water safety:

In the mid to late nineteenth century, widespread deaths from cholera and typhoid spawned a public health movement. During the early part of the twentieth century, many of the nation's larger water supply systems were installed with water treatment facilities that relied on coagulation and sedimentation, filtration, and chlorine disinfection. While these methods have been enormously effective at wiping out certain illnesses, we now face new types of microbial and chemical contaminants, which our pre-World War I water treatment systems are not prepared to handle. What's more, our water distribution system is old and crumbling;

though the water may leave the treatment plant in good order, its uncontaminated delivery to your home cannot be guaranteed.

Under development (and badly needed) are new water processing systems that involve multiple barriers to tap water contamination, including meaningful protection of source waters, installation of modern water treatment technologies (such as membranes, granular activated carbon, potentially ultraviolet radiation, and other more advanced disinfectants and treatments), and improved distribution systems.

Even if your water supply system is basically safe, keep in mind that flooding or any major emergency may make it less safe. Hurricanes and flooding can cause animal waste and polluted water to overrun normal confines and contaminate otherwise clean water supplies.

Fortunately, waterborne illnesses aren't usually life-threatening. The symptoms (fever, diarrhea, vomiting, and nausea) usually clear up within a few days. The very young, the very old, and those with weakened immune systems need to take extra care; in that case, discuss the risks with your doctor.

Nonetheless, we don't want to be drinking impure water. Here's what you should know and what you can do to keep your water safe.

## WHEN SOMETHING GOES WRONG WITH WATER FROM A PUBLIC UTILITY

Water utility companies are required to inform you if their water becomes unsafe to drink. If there are dangerous levels of microbes in your water supply, the utility company will provide instructions on how long the water must be boiled to kill the microbe. You can also buy distilled, bottled water to drink during this time.

## IF YOU RELY ON WATER FROM A WELL

- All residents who use private wells should have their water tested regularly. Extra tests are merited during extreme weather circumstances. There will be differences in the water content during a drought and during a very rainy season, and extra testing is always merited after major storms and flooding when polluted floodwaters may have contaminated well waters.
- If you are buying a home that has a well as a water source, have the water tested before purchasing. If it is a recently constructed well, the seller of the home should be able to show you certification that the well was built to code. The code for building a well will provide for protection from most types of contaminants, including normal water runoff.
- Refer to the section on pages 90 to 91 concerning testing your water for specifics on getting tests administered.
- If you are concerned about the safety of your water, boil it for ten minutes before drinking or cooking until your well is deemed safe again.
- The American Ground Water Trust is an excellent source of information concerning well water. Check their Web site or call directly: (800) 423-7748.

## POSSIBLE CONTAMINANTS AND WHAT YOU CAN DO

The biggest threats to the nation's water supply include several contaminants, none of which are systematically removed by standard methods:

*Lead:* If you have small children, have your water tested specifically for lead. Used in plumbing, lead can cause brain damage even at low concentrations. Those most susceptible to the ill effects of lead in the water are infants and children younger than age six. Exposure to the substance can cause developmental problems, learning disabilities, and lethargy.

The EPA estimates that 15 percent of the nation's households have lead in faucets, pipes, or well pumps. Those who live in older communities or houses built before 1930 are at highest risk, since lead pipes were used in plumbing at the time. Any house built before 1988, before lead laws were implemented, may have lead solder in its pipes.

To reduce lead content:

- When turning on the tap first thing in the morning, run the water for at least a minute or two before using. Lead can leach into water that has been sitting in pipes for several hours. Between uses, run the tap for 30 seconds or until the water turns cold.
- The warmer the water, the more lead it absorbs. Use only cold water when boiling for pasta, making coffee, or preparing baby formula.

***Pesticides:*** These have turned up in both well water and lakes. Children and infants—who drink more water in relation to their body weight than adults do—are at more risk from possible exposure to pesticides.

- If you live in a farming region where pesticides are used, consider switching to bottled water for children and infants from May through August, which are peak pesticide season. Pregnant women and nursing mothers may also want to take this precaution.
- If you are uncertain where the reservoir for your public utility is located and are concerned about pesticide runoff, call the utility and ask the location of the reservoir. You can also request that the company send you the latest copy of their testing report. (See the following section, "Getting Your Water Tested.")

*Chlorine:* The very substance used to cleanse our water isn't good for us in high quantities and under certain circumstances. Water companies are constantly adjusting the amount of chlorine, depending on the level of microbes in your water. Experts agree that drinking chlorinated water in limited amounts is unlikely to cause any harm. However, there may be some risk of higher incidents of bladder and rectal cancers from consuming by-products that are created when chlorine is added to the water. To reduce your exposure:

- Some of the damaging chlorine by-products are inhaled, usually when showering. Turn on the vent fan or open a window in the bathroom.
- Let water stand in an open pitcher in your refrigerator for a day or two before mixing punch or lemonade. This will evaporate most chlorine by-products and rid water of its chlorine taste.

*Chemicals:* While industrial chemicals (benzene, TCE, PCBs) can seep into groundwater from factories and industrial waste sites, they are less a danger today than they were in the past.

- If you are concerned about a particular site in your area, call the Agency for Toxic Substances and Disease Registry in Atlanta (404-639-0700).

## GETTING YOUR WATER TESTED

Unless your water source is a private well or you need to check for lead from your pipes, you don't usually need to arrange for water testing. That information should be available to you as a customer of a public utility. Request that your water company send you the latest copy of its testing report. All public water systems are now required to test for contamination and report the results to state or federal authorities. When you receive the report, the EPA allowable limits of each item will be listed alongside the contaminant. Check to see that your measurements are below the EPA levels. If the report doesn't include these limits, get a list from the EPA (800-426-4791).

If you're not satisfied, your state health department can provide you with the names of state-certified independent laboratories that can test for common contaminants. (Don't rely on testing data from water filter companies; they have a vested interest in proving your system has a problem.)

Before arranging to have your water tested, it's important that you talk to local health authorities about particular dangers in your region. It is virtually impossible to test a water sample for every type of chemical or bacterial contaminant, so you need to know what the most likely contaminants are in your area. Consider, too, your specific neighborhood. If you are within a half mile of commercial territory, you will want to test for a whole range of possibilities that wouldn't be necessary otherwise. Or if you're near a farm where pesticides are used regularly, you'll want to check for a host of other elements.

Taking a sample must be done precisely. Follow the instructions from the lab carefully, or arrange for someone to take the sample for you.

If you learn that you have a higher than acceptable level of a particular contaminant, install a water filter.

## HEALTHY WATER

Nutritionists have found that hard water (water with minerals such as calcium and magnesium, among others) may reduce your risk of heart disease. Hard water is wearing on appliances and prevents soaps from sudsing as well as with soft water, but a water softener can be added to the pipes that feed your appliances, letting you continue to benefit from the health aspects of drinking hard water.

## WHAT ABOUT BOTTLED WATER?

With the exception of distilled water, most bottled water is only slightly more pure than municipally supplied tap water. Distilled water kills cryptosporidium and other microbes and is particularly safe—that's why it's used for washing contact lenses. Some types of bottled water taste better than tap because bottling companies use ozone rather than chlorine to disinfect their water. Ozone leaves no taste or odor, but it's rarely used in public water systems because its effectiveness wears off when the water is exposed to air.

If you choose bottled water, make sure the company is a member of the International Bottled Water Association (IBWA), a trade group that monitors the quality of the water its members produce. 800-WATER-11.

## BUYING THE RIGHT WATER FILTER

Any drinking water problem can be solved with the right filter, but no filter eliminates everything. For that reason, it's vital that you have your water tested so that you'll know what kind of filter will be best for your needs.

- Carbon-activated filters absorb or physically screen out contaminants like lead and chlorine. Some of the more recent ones can also destroy microbiological cysts like cryptosporidium.
- Water softeners remove iron (responsible for bathtub stains) as well as health-related contaminants such as radium and low levels of lead.
- Reverse osmosis systems pass water through a semipermeable membrane that traps most contaminants, including cryptosporidium and Giardia. Most RO units include carbon filters as well, but they do not remove harmful bacteria. In addition, the process flushes away several gallons of water for every gallon of water generated.

- Distillation systems heat water in one chamber and turn it to steam that is eventually condensed back into water, a process that kills bacteria and removes contaminants like lead, cysts, and arsenic. These are very effective but costly to operate.

Devices can often be installed under the sink or even in the basement. Others can be mounted on the faucet or countertop. Products will be described as filtering at the point-of-use (the sink) or the point-of-entry (where the water comes into your house).

Filters cost from $20–$1000. Changing the filter and some maintenance (with some systems) will be required. Look for devices that are certified by NSF International (an independent, nonprofit standard-setting and testing group).

## ONE TOP TIP TO TEACH CHILDREN

Don't take our water supply for granted. While you will safeguard what your child drinks for the time being, a healthy dose of suspicion is a good thing if water looks, smells, or tastes funny.

## HOT BUTTON

- Get your water tested regularly if you're on a well system; if you drink public water, request a copy of the utility's "consumer confidence" report.
- For more information, and to discuss any concerns you may have, contact your public water system. The operators may give tours of the treatment system, which might be quite interesting.
- For information from the Environmental Protection Agency, call the Safe Drinking Water Hotline: 800-426-4791.

# Waste Management

When it comes to waste management, there's good news and bad news. Since 1980, the government has spent considerable effort identifying hazardous waste sites, called Superfund sites, which were created before the dangers of dumping all types of chemical and industrial by-products into the environment were known to the public. Once a site is identified, the government turns first to the company responsible for the problem and demands that it clean up the waste. If the people responsible can't be located, the Environmental Protection Agency dips into the "super" fund to pay for cleanup.

The bad news is that the governnment isn't doing much of anything about dealing with the rest of our waste. The Solid Waste Disposal Act of 1976 is not being enforced, and despite our growing population, little is being done to adequately dispose of our garbage. Most states handle waste by landfill, incineration, or by exporting it, which simply makes it someone else's problem.

The problem with landfills and incineration is that they, too, are destroying the well-being of our usable lands and water. Your children may be playing baseball on a covered up landfill that is still leaking toxic gas, and your water may be tainted by a landfill dump in which the liner is leaking.

## LANDFILLS

It doesn't take a genius to realize that in many parts of the country we are running out of places to put our garbage. Zero Waste America, an organization devoted to the elimination of waste, toxins, and pollutants, cites these as a few of the vital landfill issues:

1. Leakage: All landfills eventually leak leachate into the ground; surface water is filtered through this contaminated soil and sometimes ends up in our reserviors.

2. Water contamination: Many landfills are located next to large bodies of water, meaning that the leakage goes directly into a community's water supply. Because the federal government allows household and industrial hazardous waste to be dumped into municipal landfills, the leachate leaking from these landfills can be quite toxic.

3. Air emissions: Since the 1940s we have manufactured thousands of highly toxic chemical products, many of them commonly used in family households, which are dumped into landfills. As these chemicals break down over time, they emit hazardous vapors, contributing to air pollution.

## INCINERATORS

Burning the garbage doesn't eliminate it, it just changes it into hazardous air emissions and toxic ash, which the EPA allows to be used as a daily landfill cover. Incinerator ash is a major source of 210 different hazardous compounds that leach into soil and water and are small enough to become airborne and inhaled.

## OUR GOAL MUST BE TO REDUCE WASTE

The 1976 Solid Waste Act mandates that states maximize recycling efforts. As citizens and consumers, we can work toward creating less waste in several ways:

1. Talk to your local government about recycling programs. Some communities are more active than others. Pushing for more recycling in your own community is an achievable goal and you will almost certainly find neighbors who are willing to help.

2. Before you throw something away, consider first whether or not it can be recycled. For example, some communities

will take other types of paper when they pick up newspapers for recycling; if you can get all your junk mail into
the recycling bin, that alone is a good start.

**3.** Reduce your family's use of items that aren't recyclable, including as many plastics as possible.

**4.** Go natural. Instead of purchasing industrial strength cleaning and household chemicals, look for natural products at
health food stores or read about creating your own mix-
tures that will do the job. Soon you'll be able to buy some
natural cleansers at major grocery stores. Listening to consumer demand, some companies are beginning to come
out with "all natural" cleaners and substitutes for products
that used to be chemical.

**5.** Write to companies about taking back (and recycling)
their own containers in what is known as "producer responsibility." About 14 states have bottle bills, and companies in these states are required to take back empty
containers.

**6.** Let your politicians at all levels of government know that
you want some attention paid to environmental issues. The
right leadership can make a big difference.

## ONE TOP TIP TO TEACH YOUR CHILDREN

Set a good example and show your children the importance
of conserving our resources. Recycle, reuse, and turn out lights.
It's their world we need to save.

# Systemic and Technological Breakdowns: What to Do in a Major Systems Outage

If entering a new millennium has accomplished nothing else,
it has made us aware of our mutual dependence and vulnera-
bility. The summer of 1999 featured major power outages in cities

across the United States, caused by a range of problems. The results were inconvenient (people spent evenings on their porch stoops trying to cool off instead of indoors in air-conditioning) and serious (scientists at Columbia University in New York City lost priceless lab data when their refrigerators failed) and disastrous (more than 50 people in Chicago died in one weekend).

There's nothing wrong with enjoying all the benefits of the modern age, but we must always remember the importance of setting up systems so that we can be independent when necessary. Consider:

- Do you have a backup system for heating your home in case your gas company fails to function? A fireplace and a large supply of firewood are a good start; a generator to run some sections of your regular heating system is also an option.
- Have you stored water in case your local utility encounters contamination or a problem with their delivery system? See Chapter Four for advice on storage and recommended quantities. Also consider investing in a water purification system—a good idea regardless.
- Do you keep an emergency stash of cash at home, in case there is a major problem with your bank? In addition, you will feel more financially secure if you:

  - keep your debt down
  - save regularly and as much as you can
  - diversify your investments. The under-the-mattress syndrome is unnecessary in our society, but don't put all your eggs in one basket.
  - make extra copies of all important documents, including anything that might be stored elsewhere on computer (contracts, insurance records, bank and stock accounts, etc.).

- In general, any major breakdown in our community systems can be handled on a personal level by the type of response described in Part One of this book. However, in addition to the advice there, remember to take these steps:

- Back up your computer files (particularly financial ones) with printed copies.
- Maintain a supply of extra food in case of emergency.
- Invest in battery-powered radios.
- Have on hand a good number of flashlights.
- Be sure you have plenty of extra batteries.

## COMPUTER PROTECTION

The key to protecting your own system involves backing it up regularly, on backup disks or tapes and also via printed copies.

In addition to maintaining the safety of your own computer, the deputy chief of the federal organization charged with protecting the U.S. infrastructure against cyber attacks encourages individual citizens to get involved in protecting the national system.

The National Infrastructure Protection Center (NIPC), located in the FBI, urges people to report cyber intrusions from both the public and private sectors. By gathering data beyond what government personnel might discover, they may be able to establish protection that keeps major systems from going down.

The NIPC can be contacted in Washington by calling (202) 324-0305, or in Los Alamos by dialing (505) 667-1212.

## ONE TOP TIP TO TEACH YOUR CHILDREN

While technology is great, remind your children that it isn't a crisis when they can't get online or their video game breaks down. Books, board games, and just sitting around talking are still perfectly viable and fun ways to spend time.

# Chapter 7

# Travel Dangers

## Introduction

Your heart may beat faster when you glance at what's in this chapter. The thought of learning to avoid or survive an airline disaster is of interest to many. Yet you almost assuredly already know which sections here are most important. Your chance of dying in an airline crash is incredibly low, yet car crashes rank as the number one cause of accidental fatalities. Please read the "Car Safety" sections carefully. They are the most important in the book.

As for train and school bus safety, some of the information in these chapters will probably surprise you.

## Air Safety

When American Airlines Flight 1420 went down in a thunderstorm in Little Rock, Arkansas, early in the summer of 1999, it was the first fatal air crash of a major airline in the continental U.S. in two years. As the jet tried to land in gale-force winds, it skidded off the runway and burst into flames. Despite the severity of the crash, only nine of the 145 people on board died.

For most people, airline crashes figure high on their list of "things that most scare me." Yet air travel is by far the safest form of travel. In 1998, the fatal-accident rate for U.S. airlines dropped to .02 per 100 million miles flown. And if you should have the bad luck to be in an accident, many of the situations—as shown by the Little Rock incident and many others—are survivable.

While part of airline safety (the mechanical aspect and the actual flying) is out of our hands, there are ways we can raise our own level of safety by being responsible passengers.

## BUCKLE UP!

In nonfatal accidents, turbulence is the leading cause of in-flight injuries to passengers and flight attendants. Each year, approximately 58 passengers in the U.S. are injured by being tossed around when the flight is unexpectedly choppy. The majority of these injuries are sustained by passengers who do not have their belts fastened when the seat belt sign is illuminated.

Protecting against turbulence is simple. Just wear your seat belt. The FAA strongly recommends that all passengers keep their seat belt securely fastened at all times.

## KEEPING SMALL CHILDREN SAFE

Children weighting under 40 pounds are safest when sitting in a certified child restraint system (CRS).

- When you buy a safety seat for your car, be certain that it's also government-approved for use on an aircraft. Certain models of car seats are too wide for coach airplane seats (those wider than 16 inches), and booster seats and harness vests are banned for use on aircraft.

- The FAA recommends:

  - A child weighing under 20 pounds should be placed in a rear-facing CRS.
  - A child weighing from 20–40 pounds may use a forward-facing child restraint.

- To be guaranteed a seat for your little one, you need to purchase a separate ticket. Many airlines now offer discounts of up to 50 percent for children under two years of age. If the airlines are certain that the flight won't be sold out, you may be allowed to use an empty seat for which you haven't had to buy a ticket, though this may be a short-lived privilege. As of 2000, the FAA is moving closer to requiring some form of child restraint system for all ages of children riding in airplanes, meaning that families will be required to purchase seats for all members of the family.
- Children in restraint seats must be placed in a window seat so that the seat won't block the escape path in an emergency.
- Ask the airline to provide assistance if you have to get to another gate to make a connecting flight. Running (or even walking) through an airport with a young child, a seat, and any other carry-on bags you may have can take all the fun out of travel.

## CARRY-ON BAGGAGE

Passengers have become increasingly impatient with waiting for their luggage to be unloaded from the cargo area, and as a result, people are keeping with them an increasing amount of "carry-on" luggage. Unfortunately, when this luggage isn't properly stowed, it's a hazard to both passengers and flight attendants. Unsecured or falling carry-on baggage causes an estimated 4000 injuries per year, according to the Association of Flight Attendants.

While the airlines have taken to monitoring what is carried on, and moving the larger items to cargo you should still be watchful of what you bring on as well as what's being stowed around you.

- Current regulations specify that the maximum size carry-on bag for most airlines is 45 linear inches (the total of the height, width, and depth of the bag).
- Heavier carry-on items belong underneath seats. While some of these bags will fit in the overhead bins, it is only common sense to try to keep heavy things down below. In a worst case scenario of an accident or a bin popping open mid-flight, it is far preferable not to have a 30-pound piece of luggage crashing down on a passenger.
- Items in overhead bins should not be stacked. When the bins are brimful, it is hazardous to open them when it's time to remove your possessions.
- Notify a flight attendant if an overhead bin near you seems overly full, or if you see a passenger putting an obviously very heavy bag up above.
- Keep your own possessions pushed well under the seat in front of you, and ask that any passenger sitting between you and the aisle be equally considerate. If you have to get out in a hurry, you shouldn't be slowed by another person's briefcase.

One flight attendant on a plane landing in Memphis after a particularly choppy flight added some levity to the situation with the following announcement: "Please take care when opening the overhead compartments because, after a landing like that, sure as hell everything has shifted around."

## AIR RAGE

The stress of travel, tight schedules, sardine-can seating, and alcohol have all contributed to an increase in incidents of what is being termed "air rage," or put another way, unruly passengers. Uncooperative passengers have fondled and bitten flight attendants, yelled, thrown things, and threatened (and worse) when not given what they felt was their due—anything from another drink to the seat they wanted. Some have refused to come out of the lavatory in preparation for landing because "they were otherwise engaged," and others have even started to open emergency doors in mid-flight.

On some airlines, personnel have been granted the right to physically restrain these passengers until a safe landing can be made, and all airlines have begun taking legal action. Fines and jail time have been doled out to people who exceeded the boundaries of proper behavior.

What this means to the rest of the flying public is that at some point you may be subjected to an unruly passenger who can't stomp off in a huff. In these situations, there are a few precautions to take that will help reduce the odds of getting mixed up in the fray:

- If you are not in close proximity to what is going on, ignore it. Pay attention to your magazine and make every appearance of "minding your own business," no matter how interesting the "drama" may be.
- If the person is near you, or the person is threatening or bothering you in some way, get up out of your seat and look for the flight supervisor (the in-flight person in charge of the cabin staff), who is usually in first class. As you leave your seat, note the row and seat number of the disruptive passenger so you can identify him or her without having to do so face-to-face.
- Provide the supervisor with information about what occurred, and give him or her the row and seat number where

the person is sitting. Let the supervisor go back alone and try to calm or cope with the passenger. If there is room on the flight, you might be able to move seats.

- If you have to go back to your seat, avoid confronting the difficult passenger. You have no personal "escape hatch" on the plane, so you're better off not demonstrating any sort of emotional reaction.


## WHEN CHILDREN TRAVEL ALONE

Before booking your child on a flight alone, contact the airlines and find out about their policies regarding unaccompanied minors. Here's what you need to learn:

- ◆ If a connection is necessary, be sure your child is old enough to connect alone. Some airlines won't permit children under a certain age to be booked on connecting flights without a parent accompanying them.
- ◆ Ask about pickup on the other end. Is the airline careful about seeing the identification of the person who meets the child?
- ◆ Ask what happens to an unaccompanied child if a flight is canceled.

- Assuming that all is well and your child is booked on the necessary flight:

- ◆ Take your child onto the plane, and be certain that you're both comfortable with the situation.
- ◆ Introduce your child to the flight supervisor, and make sure he or she understands that your child is traveling without you.
- ◆ Tell your child to report any problems to the flight attendant.

- Wait to be certain the flight departs on time. Once the plane has left, call ahead to the person who is to greet your child regarding the current estimated arrival time.

## SURVIVING AN ACCIDENT

Before your palms get sweaty even thinking about the possibility of being in an airplane crash, keep two things in mind:

1. Airline accidents are very rare, and the risk of death or serious injury for air travelers is exceedingly small. Based on statistics from 1990 to 1997, Professor Arnold Barnett of the Massachusetts Institute of Technology has calculated that a passenger faces a death risk of one in eight million. Put another way, a passenger would have to choose one flight at random each day for 21,000 years before being killed in an accident.
2. Many accidents are survivable. There's no point in thinking anything else.

That said, there are some safety precautions that you can take that can make all the difference in getting out of a troubled airplane alive.

- Fly nonstop when you can. Most accidents occur during takeoff and landing so flying nonstop reduces exposure to these more accident-prone phases of the flight.
- Sit near an exit. Because every plane and every accident is different, there is no way to say that you'll be safer in the front of the plane or in the back. However, if you have to get out in a hurry, being by an exit is an advantage. Children are not permitted to sit in the emergency exit rows, but there are neighboring rows that are also quite convenient for getting out.

- As you board the flight and take your seat, locate the two exits that are closest to you. If one is blocked in an emergency, you'll need to know where else to go. Most people in airplane crashes die from the fire and toxic smoke, not from the airplane crash itself. Therefore, the most important thing is knowing how to make a speedy and panic-free evacuation.
- Because smoke can fill the cabin rapidly, count the rows between you and the exits. That way you'll be able to "feel" your way there, even if you can't see it.
- No matter how many flights you've taken, find the plasticized safety card and take a quick look at it. Experts feel that your mental preparation for reacting in an emergency is enhanced by simply taking a few seconds to focus on the fact that you might have to get out quickly. (You may have as little as 90 seconds.)
- If you're in a "worst case" scenario, the clothing you're wearing can be a help or a hindrance. Experts recommend natural fiber clothing (not synthetics), and women are advised not to travel in nylon stockings. Synthetic fabric and nylon stockings will melt onto you quickly if a fire starts.
- Keep your shoes on until after takeoff, and put them on again prior to landing. Depending on the exit method used, you may have to remove them, but for the most part, you're better off with your shoes on than off.
- Keep your seat belt fastened snugly at all times. It's your best protection from turbulence as well as impact. (The snug fit is important, because you could slip out of a loosely fastened belt.)
- Feel exactly how your belt unfastens. If the plane were to go down and you had to evacuate quickly, this knowledge would help you in getting out of your seat efficiently.
- If the oxygen mask comes down, grab it instantly and put it on, particularly if you also have to help a child. With some models, you need to tug a bit on the cord to get the oxygen flowing.

- In an emergency landing, the safest position is the "brace" position. You'll see it on the safety card in the seat back in front of you. Feet should be flat on the floor. Don't stretch your legs out. Put your arms (crossed) on the seatback in front of you, and put your head down resting on your arms. This protects you somewhat from the sudden impact that sometimes accompanies an emergency landing.

- Once the plane has landed, observe the situation. If the pilot still seems in control of the plane, wait for instructions from the flight personnel.

- If it is a crash landing, start moving you and your family toward the emergency exit as quickly as possible. Don't take *anything* with you. You may have only 90 seconds to get out. Remember your priorities: life before property.

- As you leave your seat, crouch down. In an airplane fire, your vision can be obscured by dense black smoke, and your only chance is to go low and follow the little lights on the floor to an exit. If you remember your "row count" to an exit, that will be helpful.

- Move as quickly as possible without pushing. When there is mass pushing, sometimes the exit gets so clogged that no one can get out, which is certainly counterproductive.

## TWO TOP TIPS TO TEACH YOUR CHILDREN ABOUT PLANE TRAVEL

Model these behaviors for your children so that they will think "this is just what you do" when you travel by plane:

1. Always wear your seat belt, and keep small children in child restraint seats at all times.
2. Teach them to count the rows to the nearest emergency exits. Kids enjoy activities like that, and they're great at remembering.

## HOT BUTTON

- Stow heavier items underneath seats; put lighter items in the bins above. If other passengers are endangering you because of what they put overhead, ask a flight attendant to help.
- In case of an evacuation, respond quickly and don't take anything with you.

# Car Safety

Few people realize that motor vehicle accidents are by far the leading cause of all fatal accidents, responsible for approximately 42,000 deaths and 3.5 million injuries each year. Almost 50 percent of injury deaths are car-related, according to the National Safety Council. No other single category can begin to compete with the statistics racked up by that four-wheeled everyday mode of transportation, the car.

## A SAFE CAR IS A WELL-MAINTAINED CAR

Your first protection against any kind of car mishap is to keep it in good condition at all times:

- Schedule regular tune-ups.

  - Have the car lubricated.
  - Also have checked: The brakes, steering, and wheel alignment should be examined as well as the points and plugs, the fuel emissions system and air filters, oil and oil filter, ignition wires, all belts and hoses, the windshield wipers, transmission and windshield washer fluids.

- Tires are the only contact your vehicle has with the roadway. Make sure they are properly balanced and in good condition. Depending on where you live, you may have to make seasonal tire adjustments. All-season radials may be okay if you live in a region that receives light to moderate snowfall. Even with a front-wheel drive, some areas receive enough snow that snow tires or chains are necessary.

- Have your headlight aim checked if it hasn't been done recently. One-third to one-half of all vehicles on the road have badly aimed headlights, which reduces their effectiveness for the driver and often blinds approaching drivers. (You can have them checked when your car is serviced, or you can do this yourself by loosening the two Phillips screws that keep the lights immobile and move the beam up or down and left or right. Ask someone knowledgeable to show you how the first time.)
- Cars are now being offered with internal trunk-latch releases. Because young children have died from being trapped in car trunks, General Motors developed a latch inside the trunk that is easy to use and can be seen in the dark. For about $50, GM dealers can install these devices in most of its cars engineered in the U.S. from about 1990 on. Other carmakers are putting the devices on their new models, so next time you're in the market for a new car, ask about it.

## AS A GENERAL SAFETY RULE

- Unless you're just driving around town, you should always give someone an idea of where you're going and when you'll be back.
- Someone should have the make of your car and the license number. In case of an emergency, this information gives personnel a starting point.

## EMERGENCY KIT FOR THE ROAD

Because people can go for years without ever having a problem, they get lulled into thinking that a breakdown can never
happen to them. Even if you're not handy with tools, a passenger
may be or a state patrolman who comes to your aid may be glad
you have the right equipment.

Every car should have in it the following items:

- standard pliers for holding or bending a wire (to temporarily wire up a dragging tailpipe)
- screwdrivers (Phillips and regular) for loosening or tightening a screw to correct a problem under the hood or inside
  the car
- adjustable wrench for tightening and loosening nuts and bolts
- jack
- electrical tape for fusing wiring or hoses temporarily
- light gauge wire to tie up muffler or tailpipe
- sandpaper to clean corroded battery cables
- paper towels or rags
- battery jumper cables (your owner's manual will explain
  how to use them)
- A-B-C fire extinguisher. This is only for use on a small interior fire; if your car engine ignites, get away from the vehicle as quickly as possible.
- grease-solvent hand cleaner
- empty three-pound coffee can for a variety of uses such as
  pouring water into the radiator or gasoline into the tank
- three day-night reflectors (reflectors are safer to handle
  than flares)
- extra spark plugs and fuses
- spare tire

## FAMILY AND FIRST AID SUPPLIES

Store family and first-aid supplies in a medium-size canvas bag that will conform to the space in your trunk. In it you should have the following:

- a commercial first aid kit (which should contain bandages, basic medicines, and a small first aid manual)
- distilled water to cool burns
- a blanket or two, preferably in a bright orange color in case someone is injured and must not be moved from the roadway. (Some thermal blankets can be folded quite compactly.)
- If you have children, you may want to store nonperishable food (raisins, dry cereal, etc.), water or juice boxes and some age-appropriate activity books in case you're stuck for any length of time.

## IN YOUR GLOVE COMPARTMENT

These other items should be added to the glove compartment:

- owner's manual
- a white handkerchief or piece of white cloth, to tie onto the antenna to signal for help
- a flashlight with extra batteries
- premoistened towelettes
- hand lotion

## ALWAYS TAKE WITH YOU

- your cell phone
- change for a telephone call or a phone card
- auto insurance card

- the phone number of a 24-hour tow service or your automobile club

## THE VALUE OF JOINING AN AUTO CLUB

Joining an automobile club offers benefits in an emergency.
You can call them for travel information about road conditions
(icy roads, construction, etc.), and they'll provide trip plans as
well, indicating the best roads to take. Membership can also provide peace of mind since you know that the club will send someone to your aid in an emergency. A club such as AAA has an
800-number so that even when you are far from home you can be
put in touch with a local AAA club that will see that you get help
on the highway.

## ONE TOP TIP TO TEACH CHILDREN
## ABOUT CAR SAFETY

Car trunks are very dangerous. Children should never be permitted to climb into one, even when you're standing right there.

## HOT BUTTON

- Schedule regular tune-ups for your car. A safe car is a well-
  maintained car.
- Let others know your trip plan—when you're leaving town,
  the approximate route, and when you'll be back.
- Keep your car permanently stocked with first aid and other
  emergency supplies.
- If possible, take a cellular phone with you for night driving
  or long-distance excursions.

# Vital Information about Car Restraint Systems

We wouldn't think of leaving a three-year-old on his own in the swimming pool with only an inner-tube seahorse around him. Yet every time a parent gets into a car and fails to strap a child in properly (or straps him into an improperly tethered seat), that parent is placing the child in a similarly vulnerable situation. If even a slight, near-home accident occurs, the most common kind, that child is at risk.

Motor vehicle crashes continue to lead all other causes of injury and death for American children. Each year about 600–700 passengers under age five are killed and more than 75,000 are injured as a result of vehicle collisions and sudden stops.

Providing a safe environment for your children in the car requires installing and using safety restraints properly, a task that is now mandatory in all fifty states and the District of Columbia. But it isn't as easy as it sounds. *A recent study reveals that 85 percent of car safety seats are used incorrectly.* For that reason, this section is more important than you might have guessed.

## "BECAUSE I'M THE GROWN-UP, THAT'S WHY"

First, the basics: You've got to put your child in the safety restraint *every time you get into the car together.* You've got to use a car seat on vacation (available through any car rental company), and Grandma has got to use it when her grandchild comes to visit.

Letting your child ride unbelted in the back of the station wagon or permitting a baby or toddler to ride in a passenger's lap (what experts call the "child crusher" position) for "just a few blocks" does no favor to anyone. Don't even consider bending the rules on the use of car seats and seat belts. Even when driving at low speeds, sudden stops and turns can cause injury to young ones if they aren't belted in properly. The unbelted child may injure himself by being thrown against the car's interior in case of a sudden stop, swerve, or crash, and he needs to be re-strained from being ejected from the vehicle itself. What's more, an unbelted child who is catapulted into the front seat in a sudden stop can interfere with a driver's ability to maneuver out of a bad situation.

## RIGHT CAR, RIGHT SEAT

Car safety seats are one area where you can't save money. Don't buy a used one, even as the extra seat you'll use occasionally when visiting a distant grandparents' home. With an older model, it's more difficult to know if it has been recalled, has been mistreated, is missing key parts, or has been involved in a crash. You're also unlikely to have the instruction booklet from which you can learn about installing it properly. What's more, the protective features of a car safety seat do not fully hold up after wear. Webbing of the belt system can weaken, for example.

Because of the high proportion of car seats that are improperly installed or misused in other ways, the Federal government has stipulated that as of 1999 all 100 models of car seats and all 900 models of cars should be compatible. Every child safety seat is to be equipped with two standard buckles at its base, and every new car will have standard latches in the backseat specifically designed to fasten to the buckles. By September 1, 2002, makers of car seats must also add two more straps to attach the seat bottom to a car without using its seat belt system. Automakers must equip all new vehicles with standardized attachment points for both the top and bottom straps by that date as well. Several car manufacturers will have added some of these elements before that date.

So while the new car seat you buy should be easier to use, the fact that most people will still be trying to fit the seats into older models of cars will affect their use. Before buying the seat, take a look at your car and check the instruction manual of both your vehicle and the car seat so that there will be no surprises once you purchase the seat. Make sure the seat is returnable, or ask store personnel if you can take the seat out to give it a "test fit" before making the final purchase.

While some seats purport to service infants as well as toddlers, the safest course of action is to invest in different seats:

- ***Infant-only car safety seats:*** These are designed for babies from birth to 12 months and weighing up to 22 pounds. They should be installed in the backseat of the car, facing the rear of the vehicle. Make certain that the car seat is certified for use in a motor vehicle; fastening an infant "carrier" into a car seat is not only inadequate, it's also dangerous.

- ***Convertible car seat:*** While these can be used in a rear-facing position for infants up to 20 pounds or in the forward-facing position for toddlers up to 40 pounds (about age four), the seat is rather large for an infant. If you do plan to use this seat for a very little one, roll up small blankets or towels to place on either side of the baby's body so that he or she will sit snugly within the seat.

- ***High-back belt positioning booster:*** These seats are intended for older children and are perfect for the years between toddlerhood and the size when the adult safety belt fits. These seats protect the body with a five-point harness system.

  When should you move a child to this type of booster? When he has completely outgrown his regular safety seat, which will likely be when he weighs more than 40 pounds or is too tall for it. (He is too tall if his shoulders are higher than the top set of harness slots or if the tips of his ears are above the back of the safety seat.) The booster is slightly taller and can be used with the built-in harness for children up to 40 pounds. Later it serves as a belt positioning booster.

- ***Integrated child safety seats (built into some models of cars):*** While these seats won't work for infants, they are a perfect solution to the compatibility issue between car and car seat, since no additional installation is necessary.

## WHOSE BABY IS IT?

Label your child's car seat with his or her name, date of birth, pertinent medical information, and phone numbers of adults to be contacted in the event of a major crash. If you're unconscious, emergency personnel will be able to quickly help both you and your child if this information is readily available as soon as they arrive at the scene of the accident.

## INSTALLATION

- Car seats should always be installed in the backseat.
- Never use a rear-facing safety seat in the front seat of a vehicle unless the air bag has been turned off.
- *Read the manufacturer's instructions carefully before installing any car seat.* The vehicle seat belt must be properly threaded or attached to the seat, and the seat must be secured as tightly as possible with the vehicle's safety belt to ensure safe performance in a crash or sudden stop. Some models of cars require locking clips or tethering devices, and you need to follow instructions carefully. Once the seat is in place, test its installation by pulling the base of the seat from side to side and forward. *The safety seat should be held firmly in place and should not move more than an inch in any one direction.*

The National Transportation Safety Board has asked states to set up stations where parents can have child restraints installed and checked. At this writing, only New York and South Carolina have done so, but ask around. As time passes, more and more states are likely to comply with this recommendation.

## PUTTING YOUR CHILD IN THE SEAT

Make certain the seat belt is set up adequately.

- The harness straps should be threaded through the slots so that your child's shoulders are level with or just below the strap slots, and the straps should be properly anchored. Make certain that the straps aren't twisted at any point along the way.
- The retainer clip should be at the armpit of the child's body, and it should be adjusted as the child grows.
- The straps should be tightened so that there is no more than a finger's width between the straps and the child.
- Check the adjustments periodically. The straps that have been adjusted to fit around a winter jacket will need to be tightened once a child is wearing less bulky clothing. And remember that children grow. One day you'll turn around and see that the toddler in the backseat is now quite a bit taller than she was a few months ago. The straps will need to be refit to her new size.

## ON THE ROAD

Carry a light baby blanket with you at all times. When you remove your child from the seat, toss the blanket over it. Even a winter sun can beat down on the car in such a way that the metal belts or the seat can be warm to the touch.

Before placing a child into a safety seat, check the temperature of the metal and the seat itself. If it's too hot, you may have to start the car to run the air conditioning and let it cool down before driving. Another possibility is using the baby blanket as a protective cover so that your child's skin won't touch any of the hot parts of the seat.

## USE OF A SEAT BELT

In most parts of the country, safety restraints are required for children who are under four and under 40 pounds. However, California has just passed a law that requires children to ride in booster seats or harnesses until they are seven years old.

Once your child is old enough to use a regular seat belt, here's what you should know:

- Children 12 and under should always be seated in the backseat.
- The best shoulder belts are those that are adjustable—you can change the anchor level to fit the child's height. Check the manufacturer's instructions for how to do this.
- In the rear, the center seat should have a lap belt and preferably a lap and shoulder belt.
- The lap belt should be fitted low and snugly across the child's hips—not across the stomach when he or she is sitting straight against the vehicle seat back. The child's knees should bend comfortably over the edge of the seat. The shoulder belt should stay on the shoulder and be close to the child's chest.
- The shoulder belt should *not* come across the child's face or the front of her neck. If it does, the child is not yet old enough to ride without a booster seat.
- If a child must occasionally sit in a lap/shoulder belt that doesn't fit properly, place the shoulder belt completely behind the child's back so that only the lap belt is being used. Don't use the shoulder belt under the child's arm, since this could cause serious injuries from the belt.
- Don't put more than one person in a seat belt.
- Refuse to drive unless everyone is properly fastened in a seat belt.
- Set a good example and *always* use your own seat belt.

## WHAT YOU SHOULD KNOW ABOUT AIR BAGS

As of December 1, 1998, 68 children had been killed by passenger air bags. More than 20 percent of these were with infants in rear-facing child safety seats in the front seat. An additional 70 percent were either unrestrained or improperly restrained at the time of the crash.

Although automakers are working to address the issue, and one day cars will all have air bags that can sense the size of the person riding in the seat and adjust the implosion accordingly, you need to know about today's air bags:

- With any car you buy (or already own), check what the owner's manual has to say about air bags. Some older models of cars only have air bags for the driver; others have them on both sides; still others employ side air bags. The owner's manual will contain warnings and what you need to know to protect yourself and your passengers.
- Unless you're driving a brand-new model of car with what are supposed to be safer air bags, then short adults need to sit as far back as they can from the steering wheel in order to avoid air-bag injury. If your air bag is within the steering wheel, hold your arms at 9 and 3 (o'clock positions), in order to best protect your arms in case of sudden implosion.
- Some cars now provide a manual on/off switch so that drivers can deactivate an air bag when necessary. If you simply must put a child under 12 in the front seat, you can deactivate the air bag to take away the risk of a child being injured by the air bag itself. (A light on the dash serves as a reminder to the driver and passengers that the air bag is in the "off" position.) If you buy a car with this option, check the owner's manual regarding proper use of the switch. Currently, federal requirements allow the switch only for vehicles with no rear seat or those with rear seats too small to safely accommodate a rear-facing infant seat.
- You can get authorization from the National Highway

Traffic Safety Administration to have an on-off switch installed in an existing vehicle by a dealer or a repair shop if you:

- ◆ cannot avoid placing a rear-facing infant seat in the front passenger seat.
- ◆ have been advised by a physician that you have a medical condition that places you at specific risk.
- ◆ cannot adjust the driver's position to keep your breastbone approximately ten inches from the steering wheel.
- ◆ cannot avoid situations such as a car pool that requires a child 12 or under to ride in the front seat.

- Brochures about on-off switches and installation request forms are available from local vehicle dealerships, American Automobile Association offices, state motor vehicle offices, and the National Highway Traffic Safety Administration. Switches are not available for all vehicles, so check first.

## ADDITIONAL SAFETY TIPS
## REGARDING CAR RESTRAINTS

- If you're in an accident, you *must* replace the seat. It may not be able to withstand another impact like a new one would. Your insurance company may pay for replacing the car seat. Save the receipt and show it to the insurance company. They may try to refuse, but be insistent.
- Keep the safety seat clean. Machine washing the straps and covers can cause premature deterioration of the webbing and fabric, as can the use of bleach. Follow instructions provided with the car seat, and if you have any questions, get an 800-number for the manufacturer from the store where you bought the seat.
- When traveling, always call ahead and rent a child safety seat.

- Don't let kids ride in the cargo area. Don't let kids get in the trunk—they may not be able to escape.
- Never leave children unattended in a vehicle. In warm weather they could die from heat buildup; at any time, they may figure out how to put the car in neutral or otherwise create an unsafe situation for themselves.

## SAFER CARPOOLING AND CAR TRIPS

- If you have a regular car-pool arrangement with a group, each driver should agree to the following:

  - All children should be in restraints at all times. Only permit into the car-pool the number of children that can be accommodated by the family with the smallest car.
  - Each driver should have a list of children's names, ages, and gender; a contact name in case of emergency; a photocopy of the family's insurance card; and notes about allergies or medical problems the child may have.
  - All families should agree to one pickup and one drop-off point so that the children can adjust to a routine, which will increase safety.

- To keep kids from getting fussy in their seats, take a pre-packed bag containing things to do and some car-friendly snacks (nothing that is difficult to chew, since a sudden stop could cause a child to choke on something, and nothing terribly messy so that the snacking doesn't make you irritable thinking about how everything is getting sticky). Audiotapes or CDs of children's music can be played through the car's sound system or listened to through a headset and CD or tape player. For very long car trips, consider having an adult sit in the backseat to provide amusement. Some families who take long family trips have invested in putting a television and VCR system into the car for use by backseat passengers. In addition, stop frequently for breaks.

## THE FAMILY DOG AS CAR PASSENGER

Just as a child with no seat belt is in danger of being hurt in even a minor, slow-speed accident, so is the family dog. And like an unrestrained child, a dog that is catapulted from the back of the car into the front seat can hinder the driver's ability to manage a difficult situation. For that reason, it's worth giving some thought to how you transport your pet.

- A wire partition between the back of a station wagon or sports utility vehicle and the front of the car provides greater safety for the passengers in the car and limits the distance a dog can be thrown. However, it does not provide any type of real protection for your pet.
- *Your Dog* newsletter conducted a 1999 evaluation of car restraint systems for dogs and found that the majority were useful primarily for keeping a pet under control while riding in the car, more like a leash system than a real restraint device. While such restraints can be useful, the newsletter points out that a dog could still be seriously injured wearing such a device. While product improvements will be occurring over time, as of 1999 the newsletter found only one harness system, the Ruff Rider, that the editors felt was adequate to restrain a dog in the way that a seat belt should restrain and protect a person. Watch at your pet store and look at pet-supply catalogs for new developments in this area.

## ONE TOP TIP TO TEACH CHILDREN ABOUT SAFETY RESTRAINTS

Wearing a seat belt is not negotiable.

## HOT BUTTON

- Read the instructions for your child safety seat, and make certain it's installed safely.
- Put your baby in the safety seat every time you get in the car, and make sure older kids always buckle up.

# Defensive Driving

Angry drivers, drivers on phones, daredevil drivers, drunk drivers, interstate truckers trying to stay on schedule, oversize vehicles, too many vehicles, road construction, rubbernecking—all these factors make our streets and highways more dangerous than ever before. The burden is on each of us to drive as safely as possible, and to drive *defensively*. Expect the other driver to make a mistake.

Every day you get into the car, practice driving well. The only person who can protect you is you.

## DEVELOPING THE SEAT BELT HABIT

Wearing a seat belt should be as automatic as turning on the ignition. If you're guilty of sometimes driving without your seat belt, now is the time to reform. You need to set a good example for other family members.

- Use reminder notes on the dashboard if you need to.
- Buckle up *every* time you drive.

## SAFE DRIVING: BEFORE YOU START THE MOTOR

- Daytime eye protection can actually help with night driving. Wear sunglasses whenever you're in bright sunshine (not just while driving). This will preserve a retinal chemical that helps your eyes to adapt to the dark. Too much sun exposure can reduce the ability to see at night.

- Have you just been fit with new glasses? Take into consideration how this affects your reaction time. Newly corrected nearsighted people tend to brake too quickly while newly corrected farsighted drivers tend to brake too slowly.

- If you've never been to a particular destination, plan your route in advance. If the distance is far or you have several options, contact your auto club for advice on the best route to travel.

- A key element to safe driving is being able to concentrate on the road. Children should be taught that they are not allowed to distract the driver; no playing with door handles or buttons, or sticking head or hands out the window. If children do misbehave, pull to the side of the road and explain that you're going no further until their behavior changes.

- Keep your gas tank filled. Never drive far when you have less than half a tank of gas.

- Get in the habit of locking all doors as you get in. Then the door will always be locked in case of a breakdown or a car jacking.

- While a cellular phone or a car phone is a great item to have with you in case of an emergency, don't talk and drive. Studies show that accidents increase among those who do so. There have also been news reports of pedestrians who have been killed because a driver has reached to answer the car phone, and swerved and hit a pedestrian in the process. Safety is still an issue even when using a speakerphone, probably because the driver still isn't focusing fully on the road. (A few communities are beginning to ban the practice of phoning and driving.) If you must make a call from the road, pull over at a safe stopping place or have one of your passengers make the call for you.

## GENERAL SAFE DRIVING TIPS

- Drive with your headlights on during the day. Even in bright sunshine, your headlights still make it easier for other drivers to see your car. According to a spokesperson for the AAA, this practice cuts daytime two-vehicle collisions by 30 percent.
- Use low beams in fog or snow. High beams will reflect more off fog and snow, creating more glare.
- When blinded by the high beams of an oncoming car:

  - Switch your own lights to low beam.
  - Reduce speed.
  - Look to the right edge of the pavement and use it as a guide until danger has passed.

- If the sun is behind you and low, turn on your lights. It won't improve your own visibility, but it will help others see you.
- Whenever you're unfamiliar with the roads, slow down and allow more following distance, particularly if you're behind a large truck or recreational vehicle.
- Be aware of your own blind spot as well as others'. Most cars have a spot on either side of the car that is out of range of the rearview mirrors and difficult for the driver to see without a quick turn of the head.
- Always have an alternate plan. Where would you go if something happened immediately in front of you?
- If it's wet out, be careful of hydroplaning, when water on the road is deeper than the tread of your tires. If the car ahead of you leaves no tracks, that can mean trouble. Reduce speed immediately.

- When you come upon bikes and other two-wheelers, here's what to do:

  - Lengthen your distance behind them to provide an extra margin of safety.
  - Make an extra check for them, since they can hide in your blind spot.
  - When making a right turn, be careful that no two-wheeler is sneaking up on your right behind you; they'll run into you when you turn.

- Drivers of smaller cars need to:

  - Keep a firm grip on the wheel at all times because strong winds can cause the car to swerve.
  - Know the bottom clearance of the car. Small cars may not make it over big branches, for example.
  - Make certain the car can be seen by others; use your lights and avoid getting in others' blind spots.

## NIGHT DRIVING

- Clean lights and a clean windshield make night driving easier.
- Ninety percent of driver reaction is dependent on vision. When you come out of a lighted building, it takes a few minutes for your eyes to adjust to the dark. A two- to five-minute wait can pay off in greater safety.
- Use low beams if there are lots of drivers around.
- Reduce speed at night, and increase following distance, because you need more time to react.
- Look beyond the lighted area and try to pick up hazards before you are on top of them.
- If you see a deer or other animal crossing the road, your safest course of action is to switch headlights to a lower

beam and sound your horn. Try to avoid hitting the animal; it can be very dangerous for you even inside a car.

- Never stop on the roadway at night. Other cars may drive into you, not realizing you've come to a halt.


## SAFE HIGHWAY DRIVING

- Take frequent breaks, and if possible, alternate driving responsibilities with another driver. Studies show that 56,000 accidents were caused this year by drowsy drivers, resulting in 40,000 injuries and 1500 deaths.
- On the highway, always drive with an "island of safety" around you. Use the three-second rule:

  - When the driver ahead of you passes a fixed object, such as a tree, telephone pole, underpass or billboard, start counting—one thousand one, one thousand two, one thousand three.
  - If your car reaches that fixed object before you finish counting, you're following too closely for high-speed driving. Widen the protective gap. Ease up on the accelerator. Leave extra seconds when the lighting is bad, when the road is rough, or the weather is bad.
  - If traffic has created congestion on the highway, you still want to maintain an island of safety. While the three-second rule doesn't apply to slow-moving traffic, you still need space around you to avoid hitting another car or being hit yourself in stop-and-go traffic.

- Keep scanning the scene 20–30 seconds ahead of you. On the highway this is about one-third to one-half mile or six to seven cars in advance of you.
- Drive slightly to the left of the middle of your lane so that you can see ahead.

- Watch out for cars on the roadside.
- If a truck is on your tail, move to the right lane if possible to let him pass you. If you're in the right lane, then put on your emergency flasher. This should signal to the driver that you're not going to speed up to suit his convenience. He should slow down if he can't get around you.

## IN HEAVY TRAFFIC

- Be ready to stop suddenly.
- Don't get boxed in.
- Expect the unexpected.
- When being passed, reduce your speed to help the driver get around you. That way if the person has to cut in unexpectedly, you're out of the way.
- Always expect the other drivers to try to squeeze you out of the picture.
- When approaching an intersection, slow down and look both ways, even if the signs and signals are in your favor. Be ready to take evasive action, especially at night.

## ROAD RAGE: PROTECTING YOURSELF

When the American Automobile Association Foundation for Traffic Safety studied more than 10,000 incidents of violent aggressive driving committed between 1990 and 1996, it found that at least 218 people were killed and another 12,610 people were injured, all because drivers got angry.

The AAA also conducted a study of what type of person is likely to commit road rage. According to the AAA, they are between the ages of 18–26, males, poorly educated with criminial records, histories of violence, drug use, or alcohol problems who may have suffered an emotional or professional setback. Clearly you want to avoid being a victim:

1. ***Don't offend.*** A few specific behaviors particularly enrage these angry drivers and cause them to go after you:

   ◆ *Don't cut off another driver.* Use your turn signal, check to see that there's enough space. If you make a mistake, try to signal to the other person that you're sorry (mouth the words "sorry" or use some type of body language to indicate that the other driver has the right of way). If someone cuts you off, slow down and give them room to merge into your lane.

   ◆ *Don't drive slowly in the left lane.* Even if you're driving the speed limit, don't anger those behind you. Change lanes and let them go by. Many states and provinces reserve the right lane for travel and the left for passing. If you're blocking the left lane, and the other drivers choose to pass you on the right, you've forced them to break the law.

   ◆ *Avoid tailgating.* If you are being followed closely, pull over and allow the other driver to go by. (If you can't see another driver's headlights in your rearview mirror, he's too close.)

   ◆ *Avoid obscene gestures or giving the other driver a "dirty look."*

   ◆ *Be courteous.* Signal when you're merging or changing lanes. Try to avoid using your horn; even a friendly toot can be misinterpreted. Don't fight over parking spaces and take a "be my guest" attitude toward being first, etc.

   ◆ *Don't take traffic problems personally.* No matter how angry you are at the driver in front of or behind you, you're not likely to see him ever again.

2. ***Don't engage.*** You can protect yourself by refusing to become angry at offensive drivers. Cool down. Steer clear. Give angry drivers lots of room. Don't pull over and try to "settle things." Give them space and try to get away.

3. ***Avoid eye contact.*** This makes it personal.

4. ***Get help.*** If you think you're being followed, don't go home. Use your cell phone to call for help or drive to a place where there are people. Once you're in a public area, flash your lights or honk your horn to attract attention. Don't get out of the car.

5. ***Adjust your attitude.*** Forget about "winning." Driving isn't a contest. Allow more time for your trip. Often people get upset when something slows them down. Listen to soothing music; practice relaxation; listen to books on tape—anything that makes the time pleasant.

## AVOIDING THE DRUNK DRIVER

Here are some of the facts about drunk drivers:

- Alcohol is the largest contributing factor in fatal motor vehicle accidents.
- There are approximately 2 million alcohol-related accidents annually that produce between 23,000 and 26,000 fatalities and 300,000 seriously injured victims.
- These accidents usually happen in the late evening and early morning hours, most often on weekends.
- Young drivers between the ages of 16 and 24 are involved in more than one-third of all alcohol-related traffic accidents.

To avoid being the victim of a drunk driver:

- Never get in a car with someone who has been drinking.
- Watch for all forms of erratic driving, such as wide turns, straddling the center line, weaving, swerving, drifting, slow response to traffic signals, braking erratically, excessive or very slow speed, or stopping without apparent cause, driving with head out of window, or driving with the window down in cold weather.
- If you observe any of these signs and the driver is ahead of

you, maintain a safe following distance. Don't try to pass because he or she may recover and swerve into you.

- If the driver is behind you, turn right at the nearest intersection and let him pass.
- If the drunk driver is coming toward you, you want to avoid a head-on collision between the two vehicles—the deadliest of crashes. Slow down quickly while moving to the right and stop. Sound your horn or flash your lights if there is time.
- If you see a drunk driver and can stop to use the phone, or have a passenger phone for you, call the police with a description of the vehicle, vehicle license, location of the vehicle, and the direction it was traveling. In most cases you will not need to identify yourself.

## TRAINS ALWAYS HAVE THE RIGHT OF WAY

Though there were 3,508 collisions involving a train and a vehicle or a person in 1998, these highway-rail accidents are rarely discussed. Such incidents can result in injuries and fatalities to those in the vehicle, and in almost all cases, they are caused by carelessness on the part of the vehicle driver. Operation Lifesaver, a nonprofit, nationwide public education program dedicated to reducing these accidents, offers these driving tips for intersections where the roadways meet railways:

- Never drive around lowered gates. It's illegal and deadly. If you suspect a signal is malfunctioning, call your local law enforcement agency, the railroad, or dial 9-1-1.
- Never race a train to the crossing. Even if you tie, you lose.
- Do not get trapped on a crossing. Only proceed through a crossing if you are sure you can cross all the tracks.
- If your car stalls on a crossing, get out of the car immediately, and call your local law enforcement agency for assistance.

Only attempt to restart the car if you can post lookouts to warn of approaching trains.

- When crossing multiple tracks, watch for a second train.
- Expect a train on the track at any time. Trains don't follow set schedules.
- Trains can't stop quickly. It can take a mile or more to stop once the emergency brakes are applied. Once the engineer sees you, it is already too late to avoid a collision.
- A train's large mass makes it nearly impossible to accurately judge its speed and distance.

## DRIVING IN REMOTE AREAS

If you're going to be traveling through a sparsely populated area, invest in a CB radio or a mobile phone. Not all cell phones will work in certain parts of the country, so describe your needs to the cell phone service provider to be certain your phone will work when you need it to.

- Set up a check-in system with a friend or relative. Tell them your route, the make of your car, and the license number. Also tell them your anticipated arrival time. If they don't hear from you by a certain time they should be instructed to call the state patrol.
- While driving through remote areas, make mental note of the odometer reading as you drive past homes or small towns. If you should have a problem, you'll have a rough idea whether you're one mile or 25 miles away from help.
- If you have a breakdown, staying with the car is your best option. If you do leave, everyone should go together— including small children.

## WHAT TO DO IF YOU HAVE TO PULL OVER

If you sense that something is going wrong with the steering or the engine or you see smoke, steer the car into the lane nearest the shoulder so that you'll be in a position to get off the road if necessary. If you have a choice, select a "safe haven" for your stop—the widest place on the road or an open stretch where you'll be seen easily. Get as far off the road as possible without driving into a ditch.

If you have any concern about fire, get everyone out of the car immediately, and guide them to an off-the-road spot away from the car. If the engine catches fire, there will be a lot of heat and flames.

If there seems to be no immediate crisis, then your next priority is making certain you're seen by oncoming cars. Turn on your emergency flashers and get out your warning triangles, placing one near the car and the other farther down the highway so that drivers see your warning soon enough to slow down. (If you've had to stop on the other side of a hill or a curve, place a triangle on the far side so drivers are forewarned that there is a problem on the other side.)

To notify other drivers that you need help, use the universal signals: tie a white cloth on the radio antenna or the driver's door handle or lift your car's hood.

If your car is well out of danger of being hit by oncoming traffic (easily visible and well off the roadway), then the safest place to wait is in a locked car with a window or two cracked for fresh air.

If someone other than a uniformed police officer stops, roll down the window only enough to ask them to telephone the police, your auto club, or the service station.

## ACCIDENT AVOIDANCE

- While steady pressure on antilock brakes will bring your car to a halt in the best manner possible, try to give your brakes a tap or two in the process. This will activate your brake lights, and the flash of two of the lights increases the likelihood that the drivers behind you are aware that you must stop suddenly.
- To get out of a skid, don't slam on the brakes. Quickly turn the wheel in the direction of the skid. This maneuver should let you right the car.
- Steer away from trouble. At speeds above 30 miles per hour, it takes longer to stop a car than to steer around something. In general, you're better off steering to the right to avoid a collision. If you steer to the left, you may direct your car into oncoming traffic. If it's unavoidable that you crash into something, select something yielding like a row of hedges or a snowbank. Try to stay in your own lane at all costs. If you must hit another car, it is safer for all involved to hit a parked car or one ahead of you that is moving the same direction yours is.
- If your brakes give out:

  - Pump them once or twice to see if they work.
  - If they are gone, put the car in neutral.
  - Steer into an open field, or try to find something like an open curb to rub your tires against that will help you slow down.

## IF YOU HAVE AN ACCIDENT

- The law allows you to move vehicles off the road if they are blocking traffic or are a hazard.
- Beware of leaking gas. Turn off the ignition, and don't smoke.

- Act quickly to prevent a secondary collision; put out one flare near the scene.
- Aid the injured but don't move a victim unless there is fire or another hazard.
- Call the police or the state patrol.
- You'll need the following information for your insurance company:

  - name and address of other driver(s) and license numbers of other vehicles
  - names and seating positions of other occupants
  - names and addresses of witnesses, if any
  - diagram of accident; photos if possible
  - report to your insurance company as soon as you can
  - file reports with state.

- Get the name and shield number of officer.
- If you're driving and see an accident, it can be dangerous for you. Other drivers may be "rubbernecking" (looking at the accident), and may not be paying attention to where they are driving. Always remember that gas might have been spilled and could ignite.
- If you come upon, or are involved in, a truck accident that results in a chemical spill or the release of a hazardous substance, you need to stay alert. If emergency personnel have reached the scene, they will tell people what to do; if the accident has just happened and you're not involved, try to get out of the area as quickly as possible. (Also see "Chemical Spills.")

## SAFE DRIVING: CAR JACKINGS
## AND CRIME AVOIDANCE

Most car jackings occur in early evening between 8:00 and 11:00, and mostly on weekends. Here's how not to become a victim:

- The safest type of car lock is the type with a keyless entry system. You can unlock the car when you're a few feet away and get into the car the moment you reach it.
- Always lock your doors once you get inside the car. If you have a sunroof, close it at night and in high-risk areas.
- Stay on well-traveled well-lit roads in case you need help. On your daily route, note the safe spots—gas stations, convenience stores, fire or police stations.
- Avoid high crime areas, even if it means going out of your way.
- At stop signs and lights, keep your car in gear and remain alert.
- Never leave your keys in the car when it is unattended.
- If you stop for gas, turn off your car and lock your doors when you walk over to pay the attendant.
- Never pick up a hitchhiker.
- A bump-and-run accident scam is frequently used by car thieves. When you get out to check damage, thieves take the car. If you're bumped, don't get out.
- If you're in your car and are approached by a stranger, don't roll down your windows or open your door. Honk your horn repeatedly, or use your car phone if you have one.
- If followed, don't go home. Drive instead to a safe spot. Attract attention by blinking the lights and honking.
- If you have a flat tire in a bad area, drive as well as you can on the flat tire until you get to a service station or a public area where you can get help. Sacrificing the tire is nothing compared to the risks you might run in getting out of the car.

- Cars are sometimes stolen at gun or knifepoint in parking garages, fast-food places, gas stations, and parking lots. If confronted, don't resist.

## SAFE DRIVING TIPS: PARKING

- Park in safe well-lighted areas near your destination.
- Lock your possessions in your trunk if you have one. Otherwise try to hide as much as possible from view.
- Always lock your car even for a short absence. Check inside the car before you get in.
- When you walk to your car, have your keys ready to unlock the car door.
- When possible, park on ground level in multilevel garages. Elevators and stairways can be risky.
- In an attended lot try to park near the attendant's station. Give the attendant only your ignition and car door key; never your house key. Don't tell an attendant how long you'll be—if it's more than an hour, this gives them time to use your car for foul play. When you return:

  - Check the tires to make certain they are your tires.
  - Check the odometer and gas gauge when you leave the car and when you return. Sometimes criminals siphon out gas or drive your car, returning it before you're expected back at the lot.
  - Check your license plates. Sometimes these are stolen and used in a crime.

## SEASONAL DRIVING: SUMMER

*(For information regarding winter driving, see "Winter Storms." For information regarding driving in heavy rain, see "Lightning and Severe Thunderstorms.")*

- The greatest cause of summer breakdowns is overheating. The cooling system of the car should be completely flushed and refilled every 24 months, and the level, condition, and concentration of the coolant should be checked periodically.
- Have your air conditioning system checked. A marginal system will fail in hot weather.
- Always carry two or three gallons of water (gallon milk jugs are perfect for this). Either you or your car may need water in the heat.
- Travel early (5:00–10:00 A.M.) and late (5:00–10:00 P.M.) to avoid driving long stretches during the heat.
- If your engine shows signs of overheating ("temp" or "hot" light on), stop the car and check your owner's manual for instructions. If you see steam escaping from under the hood, turn off the engine and get out of the car immediately.

## ONE TOP TIP TO TEACH CHILDREN ABOUT CARS

Cars can take the family to wonderful places, but getting to go to those places involves good behavior on the part of all passengers.

## HOT BUTTON

You are in more jeopardy when you are driving or riding in your car than you are anywhere else. Be sure to:

- Be certain everyone buckles up.
- Don't drive when you've been drinking.
- Stop frequently to avoid getting drowsy.
- Driving is an important and all-consuming responsibility.

Give it one hundred percent of your attention—no phoning and no eating. A moment's distraction can spell disaster.

# Rail Safety

If you ride a commuter train or, for longer distances, a passenger train, you're in good hands with the railroads. In the United States, rail travel of all types is a very safe method of transportation. As a passenger, you may encounter occasional delays and in a worst case scenario, a derailment, but collisions are rare, and almost any type of rail incident is survivable.

One type of accident—the highway-rail accident—usually presents little or no risk to rail passengers because of the nature of a train's braking system. Yet because such accidents can be quite serious, they get a lot of attention from the railroad industry. These accidents involve train encounters with cars, trucks, and people on the tracks. In almost all cases, the situation involves a vehicle ignoring a rail signal and trying to beat the train, or a trespasser being overtaken on the tracks by a train the person never heard coming. These accidents used to occur once every 90 minutes in the U.S., but through active work and awareness programs run by the industry and volunteer organizations, the accident statistic has dropped to once every 115 minutes. Those involved want to see the numbers come down even further.

For this reason, when it comes to rail safety, the first thing you can do to help keep you and your family safe from danger is to teach—and practice—a healthy respect for trains, train signals, and train property:

- Train crossings are well marked. When you see one, pay attention.
- If you're near a train crossing, be alert. A train can come at any time.
- If a gate is starting to come down or the signal bells are ringing to indicate an approaching train, don't ever try to

race (in a car or on foot) to get across the tracks before the train arrives. Teach your children that train signals are to be heeded at all times.

- See "Car Safety: Defensive Driving" for more advice.

If you're not in a car:

- Don't walk, run, cycle, or operate all terrain vehicles (ATVs) on railroad tracks and property or through tunnels. Despite the threat of arrest and fines for trespassing, since 1990 3,672 people have been hit and killed by trains while they were illegally on the tracks.
- Do not hunt, fish, or bungee jump from railroad trestles. There is only enough clearance on tracks for a train to pass. They are not meant to be sidewalks or pedestrian bridges.
- Don't ever attempt to hop aboard railroad equipment at any time. A slip of the foot can cost you a limb.
- At a station, don't **ever** take a shortcut across the tracks. You risk being electrocuted by the high-voltage third rail or being hit by a train. Cross to the other side of the tracks by means of an access bridge or tunnel.

## TRAVELING SAFELY BY TRAIN

As in so many situations, rail safety gained national attention several years ago because of a tragic accident: On September 22, 1993, at about 2:45 A.M., barges that were being pushed in dense fog by the towboat *Mauville* struck and displaced the Big Bayou Canot railroad bridge near Mobile, Alabama. At about 2:53 A.M., Amtrak's "Sunset Limited," en route from Los Angeles, California, to Miami, Florida, with 220 passengers on board, struck the displaced bridge and derailed. The three locomotive units, the baggage and dormitory cars, and two of the six passenger cars fell into the water. The fuel tanks on the locomotive units ruptured, and several cars caught fire. Forty-two passengers and five crew members were killed, and 103 were injured.

When the National Transportation Safety Board Railroad-Marine Accident Report was filed, it acknowledged the particulars that made this emergency extremely difficult to manage—dense fog, area accessible only by rail, water, or air, etc. Nevertheless, the NTSB did find that there was not an effective system in place to apprise passengers of train safety features. Passengers were slowed during evacuation by the absence of emergency lighting on the passenger cars, and emergency personnel were hindered because there was no passenger and crew list.

As a result of these findings, many changes have been put into effect to make trains safer and to develop better emergency procedures.

As with any other type of public transportation, it's important to board the train with the thought of keeping safety in mind.


## AT THE STATION

Some passenger mishaps occur even before a passenger has boarded the train.

- Both when arriving at the station and when getting off the train, be aware of outside weather conditions. If it's wet or snowy, the walkways may be icy. Take care as you walk.
- Listen for announcements about the train schedule; don't lean out over the edge of the platform to see if a train is coming.
- Never stand at the edge of a platform. Trains often pass through stations at high speeds, and the resulting air turbulence can cause you to lose your balance.
- Never leave children unattended in stations or on icy platforms. Hold the hands of small children, who may not realize the care that is necessary when standing on a train platform.

- Due to track maintenance or emergency situations, sometimes a temporary bridge provides the only access to getting on or off the train. These bridges can be particularly slippery, so wait until the train has come to a complete stop before stepping onto the bridge plate, and always use handrails.
- Never take a shortcut across the tracks.
- Assume that a train may be coming at any time.

## BOARDING AND DETRAINING

- Trains and platforms don't always meet up evenly at every stop, and there will always be a gap. As you board or exit a train, be sure to watch your step. Handrails can be a help.
- Don't stand in the vestibule (car ends) when the train is moving. Enter these only when you have to pass between cars. Never ride between cars, and during the winter months when it can be icy or slippery, try to avoid moving from car to car.

## ON THE TRAIN

- Just as in plane travel, when you board, note emergency information, which is now provided on long-distance passenger trains either in the seat backs or in posters located on the walls of the car.
- Take a moment to familiarize yourself with the passenger safety information card. Note the locations of the emergency windows, and take a moment to read how to operate them.
- On a passenger train, every car will have at least one well-marked emergency box containing a first aid kit and snap lights, which can serve as emergency lighting if the power on the train should fail. Locate the emergency box as you get on.

- Stay in your seat as much as possible. If you must walk through the train, use one hand to steady yourself by holding on to seat backs or the edge of overhead luggage racks. There are handrails to use in the restroom.
- Always wear shoes when you leave your seat. Floors can be slippery, and there are metal plates on the floors between cars that can move and injure bare feet.
- In an emergency, remain calm and wait for announcements as to how to proceed. In most cases, you will be instructed to remain on the train. If personnel do want you to disembark, it will be important to learn whether they plan to evacuate passengers out emergency exits or by walking from car to car to get to an end.
- If you are to leave the train, assess the outside conditions before exiting. Once out, move away from the tracks.
- Offer assistance to the elderly, disabled, or others in need.
- If you see a fire on the train or in a station, immediately inform a station or train employee. If there is a fire or smoke in your car, immediately move to the next car.

## THREE TOP TIPS TO TEACH YOUR CHILDREN ABOUT RAIL SAFETY

1. Teach your children never to trespass on railroad property.
2. Don't ever let them talk about "racing the train" at a crossing.
3. When traveling with your children, demonstrate safe behavior on the platform and on the train.

## HOT BUTTON

- Trains always have the right of way. Take crossing signals seriously.
- Pay attention to safety when getting on and off the train. Platforms can be slippery in inclement weather.

- An aware passenger is a safe passenger. As you board a train, read any safety information that is available, and locate the emergency box in your car.
- Keep track of children at all times.

# School Bus Safety

Traveling by school bus is actually a very safe method of transportation, with an average of only nine deaths per year. But what parent can tolerate "only nine"?

That's why there's still so much interest in school bus safety. Once a child is placed on a school bus, parents, school officials, and the community all want to make sure that each and every one of those kids arrives home safely.

## WHY NO BELTS ON BUSES?

Seat belts on school buses made big news in 1999 when the National Transportation Safety Board announced that they recommended more padding around seats rather than the addition of seat belts to school buses.

School buses built since 1977 rely on closely spaced seats with high, padded seats for protection, a method that is known in the bus industry as "compartmentalization." Studies have shown that a lap belt is exceedingly dangerous because by holding a child's pelvis firmly in place, it allows the torso to snap forward and back with the possibility of a child's head hitting the seat back with more force than if the child's whole body had been thrown. Lap and shoulder belts together offer some improvement, but because the sideways shift in bus crashes is much greater than the sideways impact in a car accident, a child's shoulder is easily shaken loose from the shoulder belt, and the dangers of the lap belt take over.

Nonetheless, an understandable parental complaint about

this system is that it lets kids get out of the habit of fastening a seat belt every time they get into a vehicle.

School bus safety is far from a closed topic. What will eventually come to pass will likely be the redesign of the seats to include armrests, ceiling pads, and molding the seats and seat backs to the human form so that the seat is more successful at cushioning high impacts.

## SAFETY BEGINS AT THE BUS STOP

The greatest number of accidents involving children and school buses actually take place around what is known as the "danger" zone, the area in the immediate vicinity of the bus.

First, check your child as he or she leaves in the morning. Make sure there are no loose or dragging drawstrings or ties on his clothing or backpacks. Only recently, a child's drawstring got caught as the door closed when she was getting off the bus. She was pulled under the bus and killed before anyone realized what had happened.

Stress to your children the importance of safe behavior around the bus stop:

- Arrive at the stop at least five minutes before the bus is due to arrive, so that there's no rushing in front of traffic to get onto the bus.
- Children should wait for the bus at the designated loading zone. If you pick your child up afterward and are running late, tell him to wait there after school as well.
- Once on the bus, children should be taught not to distract the driver. They should remain seated, keep the aisles clear, and keep their arms and hands inside the bus. They should not throw things.
- When boarding or leaving the bus, children should wait until the bus comes to a complete stop, then walk in a single file to the front of the bus, and get off using the handrail.

- Point out to your child that the driver has a blind spot approximately ten feet wide directly in front of the bus. Children must be very careful when they walk in this area. Tell them that if they must cross the street after getting off the bus, they should do so at least "ten giant steps" in front of the bus.
- If a child drops anything around the bus, she shouldn't stop to pick it up. Instead, return to the bus and ask the driver for help. If a bus monitor is available, she can supervise retrieval of the item and signal to the driver when it's safe to proceed.

## HOT BUTTON

- Have your children review all these safety measures with you. You can't always be with them, and it's vital that they understand how important bus safety is.

## Chapter 8

# Public Dangers

## Introduction

A stampeding crowd, a stalled elevator, a personal attack of some kind, and school violence—these are the types of issues out of which nightmares are made. The statistical odds of you or a family member being caught in any one of these situations is very low, but if it ever were to happen, this is what you would want to know.

## Crowds

Few things could be worse than being caught up in an uncontrollable crowd, unable to free yourself from a crush of humanity. People can be badly hurt and even killed when they aren't able to extricate themselves from a crowd.

### WHAT CAN HAPPEN

British soccer fans have experienced some of the worst "crowd tragedies" of recent years. In Sheffield, England, in 1989, thousands of fans were at a soccer stadium to see Liverpool play Nottingham Forest in an important qualifying game. As the game started, Liverpool fans were still trying to get into the stadium. Intending to relieve the crush at the fence, the police unlocked another gate and the supporters came flowing in. But the stands were already packed. As the crowd grew, people in the front of the stand were crushed against the fence between the spectators and the field.

Six minutes into the game, the referee called a halt, but people still kept pushing toward the field. By the time someone thought to open the gates and permit people to spill onto the field, 96 fans had been crushed to death and more than 200 others were injured. (Four years before this, Liverpool fans had charged the stands at another game, and 35 people died in that tragedy.)

But Britain is by no means alone in such incidents. Probably the worst one in recent U.S. history was the 1979 Who concert in Cincinnati, when eleven rock fans were crushed to death and scores were injured.

## WHAT TO DO

Here's what you need to know to protect yourself in a situation where "pack mentality" may rule:

- Anytime you enter any large environment—a stadium, a theater, a mall—always know how you would get out if you needed to. Where are the exits? What path will you take to get there?
- How and where you are can also make a difference in the level of safety. At games and concerts, standing room only, festival seating, or general admission tends to be the most dangerous. While it can be fun to be amid an enthusiastic crowd, it can easily get out of control.

- Practicing "situational awareness" is vital in such circumstances. Attend games, go to concerts, watch parades, but always pay attention to the mood of the crowd. If you begin to sense an unruliness, or if one or two individuals start acting up, start moving out of the crowd. Timing is everything.
- Consider the group that makes up the crowd. Enthusiastic as they are, opera fans tend to be more contained than, say, football or hockey fans. If you're outside the Metropolitan Opera House at New York's Lincoln Center in a big crowd, you're not likely to be swept up by a group pushing toward the door. But if you're at a hockey game or a band concert, particularly if there has been a lot of drinking or the use of illegal substances, pay attention to what's going on around you. An unruly crowd that is well-filled with alcohol is more difficult to manage than a sober one.
- No matter how great the concert or how terrific the game, if there's going to be trouble, you'll want to get out when you can. Leave early if you have to. Or if the unruly ones are pushing toward the exit, hang back in a safe location and wait until the crowd thins out.
- If a crowd is already beginning to surge behind you, sidle sideways to get out of the crowd. If you can't get to either side of the crowd, look around for some type of architectural structure and stand so you are protected from the crush.
- If you are knocked down, assume the fetal position and cover your head until the crowd passes by.

## THREE TOP TIPS TO TEACH CHILDREN ABOUT CROWDS

1. Children should have identification on them at all times. This is particularly important in a situation in which you could be separated. If the kids are teens, they should have their name on them somewhere anyway.

**2.** In big crowds, pick up young children. A sea of people is frightening enough. Imagine seeing only a sea of legs.

**3.** Teach crowd awareness. Rock-concert-age kids must keep their wits about them. Teach them to sidle out of the center of any big group that begins to make them nervous. Even kids get spooked by these things.

## HOT BUTTON

- Maintain a high level of "situational awareness" in crowds. Try to realize ahead of time that you don't want to be in the midst of this group when it starts to move.
- If you're a little late in realizing you have a problem, try to keep edging sideways to get out of the middle of the crowd.

# Elevators

How many times have you been in an elevator, only to have it come to a sudden halt with you thinking—"Is this it? Is this the time the doors don't open?" Or have you ever entered an office building or a hotel lobby and heard the alarm bells sound, thinking: "Thank goodness it's not me."

Elevators do get stuck occasionally, but the good news is they are relatively safe to be in even then. The units in place today have more than one form of safety cable, and if anything should go wrong, there are guide rails to keep the elevator from swaying from side to side and a brake system to keep the elevator from going into free fall.

Though no one keeps records of elevator accidents, an estimated 6500 people go to the hospital for elevator-related injuries each year. Most commonly people are struck by closing doors, or they trip and fall getting out of the elevator when the floors aren't even. Although there have been more than 100 deaths since 1991 from elevator accidents, almost all were preventable.

So long as you remain calm and use common sense, the chances are quite good that you'll be perfectly safe no matter what happens in an elevator.

## GENERAL SAFETY TIPS

- Don't rush to pry open a door.
- Pass up an overly crowded elevator.
- Make sure the floor and elevator are even when getting on or off.
- When the elevator door opens, make sure the elevator is there. Every now and then the doors open, and there's no car.
- Don't lean on the doors. Most elevator accidents involve malfunctioning doors.

## IF YOU GET STUCK

- Once you realize the elevator has stopped, your first task is to ascertain whether you're stuck between floors or whether the doors simply didn't open. Try pushing some of the buttons, including the "open door" button. If nothing happens, then let others know you're stuck.
- Look for the telephone or headset systems that are available on most elevators. Use it to call out if you can. If not, try the alarm. If you or someone who is stuck with you has a cell phone, use it to call 9-1-1. Tell the person who answers the building's address, and if you know the elevator bank or can find an identification number in the elevator, provide that information, too. If you know between which floors you're stuck, rescue personnel may be able to get you out faster.
- Don't ever try to climb out of a stalled elevator. You risk falling into the shaft. At least a dozen people have died this

way. When people jump out of a car and down to the landing, they sometimes lose their balance and fall backward.

- Despite what you see in the movies, never climb on the roof
  of the elevator car.
- If you're lucky, the company or hotel will stay in touch with
  you until you're rescued. At one hotel, personnel even
  brought orange juice to the guests who were stuck.
- Sit on the floor and wait for help. If you must stand, hold on
  in case the elevator starts up unexpectedly.
- Stay calm. Sometimes people panic after a certain period
  of time and decide to jump out. Don't. Instead, calm down
  and wait—even if it takes 40 hours to be rescued, as it did
  one man in New York City, in the fall of 1999, who tried to
  leave work on a Friday evening and remained stuck in an
  elevator until Sunday night.

## ONE TOP TIP TO TEACH YOUR CHILDREN ABOUT ELEVATORS

If you get stuck, use one of the communication systems to call
for help. Someone will come to get you out.

## HOT BUTTON

- Remain calm. Don't try to climb out or pry the door open.
  Sit down and wait for someone who is knowledgeable to
  arrive.

# Personal Safety

Whether it's a purse snatcher on a busy street or a crazed for-
mer employee who returns to the job, there are two basic rules to
follow in keeping yourself safe:

1. Remain "aware of your situation" at all times. In Emergency Manager Randy Duncan's introduction, he addresses "situational awareness." Whether you're in a car, at work, or walking along a street, you've got to pay attention. At times, your life will depend on it.
2. Avoid trouble. Don't invite danger by acting contrary to common sense. Reduce your risk by avoiding dark streets and by parking in well-traveled areas at night. Keeping your wits about you offers the best self-protection. In addition, the National Self Defense Institute offers these guidelines:

## AT HOME

- Keep your windows locked, and lock the door behind you as you enter.
- Install a peephole in your door and use it.
- Close your drapes and blinds, to keep your movements private and your possessions less conspicuous.
- Light your yard and garden well so that criminals don't have dark places to hide.
- If you move to a new home, change the locks right away.
- Let your building management (or the police) know if unauthorized people are hanging around your neighborhood.
- Call the police if you hear strange noises or see something that alarms you.

## WHEN COMING AND GOING

- If you can, vary the times you leave and return home each day.
- Leave a dim light or softly-playing radio on when you leave home.

- Be sure exterior lights will be on if you return after dark.
- If possible, let someone know where you're going.
- Go out with other people whenever possible. There is safety in numbers.
- Consider getting a dog.
- See "Car Safety: Defensive Driving" for safety information when you're driving or in parking lots.

## SHOPPING

- You might look like a potential victim if you're loaded down with packages. Make certain you don't carry more than you can comfortably manage and still be alert to what's going on around you.
- Consider choosing a supermarket where people will take your groceries to the car with you.
- If you're shopping with your child, don't put your child in the car before the groceries. If someone takes your car at that point, you won't want your child to be in it.

## ON PUBLIC TRANSPORTATION

- Stay awake and alert.
- Don't flash money.
- Put your money and credit cards in different pockets so that if someone robs you, he won't get everything.
- Stay in well-lit areas while waiting for a bus or a train.
- Stand back from the street or the edge of the platform. If you stand too close, you're more vulnerable to being pushed from behind.
- Ride near the train conductor or bus driver or ride with a big group of people.
- In a taxi, note the driver's name and taxi number.

## AT THE ATM

- Avoid going at night, or take a friend.
- Look for machines in well-populated areas.
- Keep your card, your deposit, and the cash you receive out of sight.
- Use your body to block others' view of the keypad and screen.
- Use any reflective surfaces as mirrors to see behind you.
- If someone does try to rob you, give up the money. Better to lose the cash than your life.

## HOT BUTTON

- Pay attention to what you're doing and what's going on around you. In doing so, you're less likely to become a victim.

# School Violence

There is no greater parental nightmare than what happened at Columbine High School in Littleton, Colorado, in the spring of 1999, or in several other schools across the nation in which students and teachers were shot, maimed, and killed. The very thought that your child might not come home from school one day is too much to bear.

In reality, your child is far more likely to witness or be a victim of a fistfight or an unpleasant taunting, also far more likely to be killed riding a bicycle, than he or she is likely to experience a multiple shooting. Still, one can't help but consider what can be done to try to prevent such violence from happening elsewhere.

There are no easy answers. The U.S. Secret Service has undertaken a detailed review of shootings at more than a dozen schools to identify motives and behaviors, to help schools and police recognize which students are likely to kill. What they have already learned from studying assassins poses a conundrum for those who are struggling to prevent school violence. Often what we hope will help "cure" the problem—surveillance cameras and armed guards, for example—actually exacerbates it. Studies show that these individuals often want notoriety above all, and they won't hesitate to die in a "blaze of glory." To a troubled person planning on violence, armed guards with the potential to kill may actually make the situation more attractive.

However, it is clear that recent student killers have some traits in common: the shooters thought others viewed them as inferior and powerless; they had easy access to, and had a special fascination for, violent entertainment; they had access to guns.

At a conference on school violence held the summer following the Columbine incident, experts also agreed on this point: That the kids involved in all the incidents were troubled children whose problems were often revealed through a lack of social skills, scant peer acceptance, and a breakdown in communication. Crises with these children occur when a buildup of emotional stress in their lives leads them to snap. As one expert says, "Water doesn't suddenly boil; it builds up to it."

Because identifying children who have the potential for violence is not an exact science, we as parents must do what we can to find ways to safeguard our children. The best approach is to work with the two elements you know best—your child's school, and your child—to try to make your community as safe as possible.

## TALK WITH SCHOOL ADMINISTRATORS

- Don't go in demanding metal detectors and police officers in the building, but ask what the school is doing to increase safety. Each community and school is unique, and neither metal detectors nor police officers can offer ultimate reassurance that no weapon will ever be brought into school. Some schools are refusing to become fortresses; some administrators feel that extreme measures put the borderline student even more on edge. Instead, school systems are using many methods to try to avoid school violence. At your school they should be talking about two types of plans—for preventing and for responding to a crisis:

♦ **Prevention:** School administrators should discuss with teachers what to look and listen for when trying to identify troubled individuals. Depending on the school location and the makeup of the student body, schools are also opting for other preventive methods. Some are using handheld metal detectors for spot checks, finding them more effective (and less negative) than the constant presence of metal detectors at all doors. Some schools are using computerized identification cards to control access to the schools; others are requiring the use of transparent backpacks so the contents are visible to everyone.

Charleston, South Carolina, has just completed a gun-free year at the schools as a result of a new program. After determining that showing off was a prime reason why students brought guns to school, the police department started offering a $100 bill to anyone who could tell the department where they could retrieve a gun—even a toy gun—that had been brought on to the school premises. As a result, the interest among students in bringing their guns to school has diminished considerably.

♦ **Crisis Response:** Does the school have a plan for dealing with violence? Are students and administrators prepared? Police departments should have a floor plan of your school. Some schools are setting up caller-ID systems for the phones and running disaster drills with emergency personnel.

- Do ask whether the middle and upper schools in your community have been assigned their own certified law enforcement officers. When used properly, they can serve three purposes:

**1.** They work as peacekeepers, just as any police officer would do.
**2.** They work in the classroom to educate students about the law. The student who understands the difference between a misdemeanor and a felony, the one who knows the penalty for being caught with drugs, and the one who knows that an officer does have the legal right to search a locker, is far more likely to walk the "straight and narrow" than those who are ignorant of these issues.
**3.** They serve as law-related counselors, referring troubled students to resources within the community that can provide necessary help.

## SUPPORT THE SCHOOL AND WORK CONSTRUCTIVELY

- Be positive and supportive of the school in general. If your child senses your positive interest in the place where he spends most of his day, he's more likely to feel safe, work hard, and obey the rules.
- Don't help your child get around school rules. Sending in an "excuse" note on a day when a bunch of kids want to cut school for a baseball game sends a bad message that ricochets far beyond what your child misses in a couple of classes.
- Be involved in your child's school life by attending as many events as you can and talking to him or her about schoolwork and school activities.
- Work with your school to involve more parents and make the school responsive to all families.

## POSITIVE PARENTING FOR RAISING GOOD KIDS

- Give your children consistent love and attention.
- Be consistent about rules and discipline.
- Keep lines of communication open with your children and get to know their friends.
- Take your children's complaints seriously.
- Note changes in your children's behavior—a sudden shift of friendships, cruelty to others, behavior problems in school, etc.
- Make certain your children are supervised; know where they are and whom they are with.
- Encourage your children to have special interests and make time to get them to their activities. The involved and committed child is less likely to have problems of any type.
- Teach your children that violence is never an acceptable option. Don't ever hit your children. Physical punishment teaches a violent solution.
- Address violence in the media and in the community. If you didn't enjoy a movie because it was violent, say so. If something bad happens in the community, take time for the family to talk about it.
- Make sure your children don't have access to firearms, and don't carry one yourself. Violence should not be put forth as a solution, ever.

## TEACH YOUR CHILDREN TO MANAGE THEIR ANGER

Everyone needs to learn how to diffuse negative emotions. This skill is particularly important to schoolchildren because blowing up in anger at a potentially violent person may trigger a violent response.

- Help your children find constructive ways to deal with conflict. Teach them how to control and diffuse their anger (leave the situation, find a calm person to talk to) before dealing with the situation.

- Also teach them:

  - ◆ Don't lash out verbally. Verbal abuse or a flip remark can spark as much trouble as punching someone.
  - ◆ Always consider the consequences of anything you say or do.
  - ◆ Try using humor to cool hostility.
  - ◆ Never fight with anyone who is using drugs or alcohol, or likely to have a weapon.
  - ◆ Learn what you can about both sides of a dispute, and then think of solutions that will satisfy both parties.
  - ◆ Never make bias (race, religion, sex, or sexual orientation) a reason for a dispute.
  - ◆ If someone picks a fight, refuse to be pulled into it.

## TEACHING YOUR CHILDREN LIFE STRATEGIES FOR DEALING WITH THE "UNCOMFORTABLE"

We all have moments when we feel uneasy about our safety—on the street at night; in a parking garage; when we accidentally cut off another car and the driver becomes enraged. Such situations happen throughout life, and your children will encounter similar moments at school, too. Basic life strategies are necessary to stay safe in these situations. If your child encounters something that makes her feel uncomfortable:

- *Avoid the situation.* Select a different route to get to school, or stay away from the part of the playground or school property where a particular group hangs out.
- *Stay with a group.* There is safety in numbers.
- *Avoid confrontation.* Don't make eye contact; don't respond to taunts; don't say bad things to others about the

person who is threatening you. This gives the person added reason to pursue the fight.

- *Report the situation as soon as possible.* The school administration should be prepared to intervene in these situations, though your child will still need to be careful.

## TALKING TO YOUR CHILDREN ABOUT POTENTIAL CRISES

What can you do to help your children cope if they're faced with a horrific crisis? You're already doing it by making safety-consciousness a regular part of your family life. Remind your children about emergency manager Randy Duncan's "situational awareness" philosophy. The student who remains aware of his or her surroundings, and maintains the presence of mind to assess the situation, is the one who will make the right decision for him- or herself. If you've been serving as a good role model in how to handle a crisis, your child is already better prepared than you might expect.

That said, there are two points you can make to your child that might prove helpful:

1. Talk to your child about tolerance and respect for others. In the school shootings, the children involved in the shootings felt like outsiders; in the Columbine incident they were specifically tired of being taunted by the popular athletes. Teenagers are prone to putting others down in order to validate their own position, but they can be discouraged from such behavior. The more parents there are who teach against it, the safer the schools will be.

2. Talk about the importance of reporting to a trusted adult anything your child hears that involves a threat. In many of the shootings, other kids had heard the child or children in question make threats—they just didn't say anything to authorities.

## HOT BUTTON

- Get involved in your children's schools, and show support for the activities and the authorities.
- Keep the lines of communication open with your children, and take their comments seriously.

# Chapter Nine

# Food-Related Dangers

## Introduction

According to the Centers for Disease Control and Prevention, an estimated 5,000 people per year die and a shocking 76 million—more than double the previous estimate of 30 million—get sick from eating tainted foods. Keep in mind, too, that food-borne illnesses are underreported because people don't always go to their doctors for less severe stomach upsets.

There has been a recent increase in financing for food safety, partly because the government is concerned. The organisms that cause illnesses are becoming more virulent, and because more food is coming from fewer sources, there is a growing possibility that larger numbers of people than ever before could fall ill. (The days of local and regional food distribution offered the advantage of limited exposure.)

The government has set up eight sites around the country for active surveillance of food-borne disease, in the hope that they'll spot outbreaks quickly and be able to stop them.

But when it gets right down to it, we each must take responsibility for our own food safety.

# General Food Safety

While we know a great deal more about sanitation and proper food preservation and preparation than previous generations did, today's families are now more demanding. Not only do we want the option of buying everything from tomatoes to straw-berries all year round, but we also want a lot of the preparation done for us. "Triple washed" lettuce is a prime example.

These circumstances endanger us to some extent, because we're giving up control over what we eat. It's anyone's guess as to the water and soil quality wherever it is those imported out-of-season blueberries were grown. And if you've ever read about where some of that "triple washed" lettuce is washed, you'll put the next bag you buy right into the salad spinner for one good old home-style washing.

Here's some of what you need to know to protect your family.

## CLEANLINESS IS NEXT TO . . .

- Wash your hands before cooking, and throughout the process if you think you may have touched something raw or unclean. If you're wearing rubber gloves during any of the food preparation process, wash them as well.
- Mix up a cleaning solution to have on hand to disinfect surfaces as needed. Mix one part liquid chlorine bleach to ten parts water and store it in an empty bleach bottle. Keep it conveniently located but inaccessible to young children.
- Make certain all cooking surfaces and cutting boards are clean. Dedicate one cutting board for cutting up meat; the other can be for fruits and vegetables. Use the bleach solution to disinfect after use.
- Avoid cross-contamination. Don't use the same spatula to flip the uncooked hamburgers and take the cooked vegetables off the grill. Use separate utensils for cooked and un-

cooked foods; get a clean spatula when it's time to take the cooked burgers off the flame, for example.

- Always wash fruits and vegetables thoroughly.

  - ◆ Wash the exterior skins of cucumbers and the outer rinds of melons. If the skin or rind has surface bacteria and you cut through it, the knife will take the bacteria inside.
  - ◆ Use a vegetable brush on the less delicate items, and run all produce under water, washing it as thoroughly as possible.
  - ◆ Don't use soap. It actually increases the porousness of some of the fresh produce and allows bacteria to get inside.

- Don't wash the dog or cat bowl with the same sponge you use on your dishes or countertops.
- Toss your sponges into the dishwasher for cleaning, or put some of the chlorine solution in a bowl and let your sponge soak in it overnight.
- Sanitize your drain, disposal, and pipe with a solution of one teaspoon of chlorine bleach in one quart of water. Food particles get trapped and bacteria can grow.

## PROPER HAND WASHING

Washing hands before preparing food and before eating is extremely important for all family members. Experts recommend that hands should be washed under warm water with soap for approximately 30 seconds. Work the soap between fingers, under rings, and around nails before rinsing and drying them. Children should be taught to wash this way as well. Suggest that they sing one verse of "Row Row Row Your Boat" or some other simple song every time they wash their hands. That will mean that they do more than just a cursory wash.

## SHOPPING

- When running errands, make the grocery store your last stop, and put things away as soon as you get home.
- Check the "use by" and "sell by" dates:

  - The *sell by* date is the date on which the product is to be pulled from the shelves. Under proper refrigeration, most dairy products should keep for seven days once you get them home. Meats will vary depending on type and thickness. Chops, steaks, and roasts should keep for three to five days; stew meats, ground meats, and poultry for one to two days. Keep in mind that most products that have a "sell by" date are generally packaged (meats) or have arrived in the store (dairy items) several days prior to this date. The management of the store's refrigerator section may affect the condition of any food that has been around for a few days. Try to buy products with a date that indicates they've been most recently delivered to the shelf.
  - The *best-if-used-by* date is commonly used on items such as cereals and snacks. These items generally have a shelf life of more than six months, but the product is likely to taste stale as the stamped date draws near.
  - The *pack date* is used on some canned goods, as well as on some fresh fruits, vegetables, and red meats.
  - The *expiration date* is found on refrigerated dough products and packaged yeasts.

- If you buy a dated item, use it while it's still as fresh as possible; many foods can be frozen to extend the time during which you can use them.
- When shopping, avoid purchasing food that looks marginal. Ground meat packages should be cold and tightly wrapped, and the meat surface exposed to the air will be red; the interior of fresh meat will be dark. Other refriger-

ated food should be cold to the touch; frozen food should be rock-solid; canned goods should be free of cracks, dents, or bulging lids.

- Refrigerated items such as meat should be put into the cart last so as to minimize the length of time the meat is not refrigerated. However, don't place the meat packages on top of other groceries—burrow down in your cart so that the meat can be placed near the bottom where the juices won't leak out onto other things you are buying.

## KEEPING HOT THINGS HOT, AND COLD THINGS COLD

- Use a digital thermometer to determine interior meat temperatures: Ground beef and pork should be heated to 160; beef, veal, lamb, steaks, and roasts should be at least 145; poultry needs to reach 180. Wash the thermometer probe with hot water after each use to prevent contamination.
- Don't stop cooking food before it's done. Harmful bacteria will grow in partially cooked food, even if it's refrigerated.
- When cooking in a microwave oven, cover the food, stir, and rotate the dish for even cooking. Bacteria can survive in the cold portions of food. Allow microwaved food to stand for a few minutes after cooking; this distributes the heat and assures thorough cooking.
- Refrigerate leftovers promptly. Just because it is cooked doesn't mean it is safe to leave the food out.
- Keep your refrigerator at 40 degrees F or below to keep harmful germs from growing and multiplying.
- Don't thaw foods on the counter. Leave packages of frozen food in the refrigerator or use the microwave.
- When in doubt, throw it out.

## WHY DON'T YOU JUST SKIP IT?

Sushi can carry parasites, bacteria, viruses. Unless you know the supplier and how the fish was handled, it's best not to eat it. Freezing kills parasites but not viruses. Never feed sushi to anyone in a high-risk group—the very old, the very young, or anyone with a suppressed immune system.

## RESTAURANT CHECKUP

It's wonderful to be waited on (or at least not to have to cook), but you know little about how the food was prepared or who did the cooking. The best way to judge the safety of the food preparation is to check the restaurant's bathroom. If it's unclean, then that means employees may not have had a good place to wash up. Look for someplace else for your next meal.

Also be wary of salad bars. Consider the number of ways food can be contaminated. If a serving spoon—handle and all—drops into a salad, pasta, or vegetable dish, the food is contaminated by all the hands that have touched that spoon. Some kitchens reuse food that has already been out on the bar; if the tuna bowl is partially empty, the new refrigerated tuna may simply be mixed with the leftover tuna—you have no idea what you're eating. If it's your only option for a quick bite, at least check superficial cleanliness: Is there a sneeze guard (plastic shield protecting the food)? Is the staff wearing gloves? Is the produce fresh? Are the hot dishes hot? Are the cold dishes cold?

## KNOW THE SYMPTOMS OF FOOD POISONING

If someone in the family becomes ill with what seems to be food poisoning, knowing the cause can make a difference in the treatment. Here are some symptoms and what usually has caused them.

- Nausea, vomiting, and diarrhea less than six hours after eating can usually be traced to bacteria in dairy products, poultry, or meat left at room temperature or in the sun.
- Stomach problems and burning or tingling sensations of the mouth, tongue, and face within six hours of eating are symptoms of seafood poisoning.
- Fever, cramps, and diarrhea between 12 and 72 hours after eating can be the effects of an infection from eggs containing bacteria, the most common of which is salmonella. (See "Salmonella.")
- Acute and possibly bloody diarrhea can occur 72–120 hours after eating undercooked hamburger or drinking unpasteurized juices, and may be caused by E. coli. (See "E. Coli.")

## ONE TOP TIP TO TEACH CHILDREN ABOUT FOOD SAFETY

Helping children develop the habit of washing their hands before meals and frequently throughout the day will not only lessen the chance that they will contaminate what they eat, but it will also cut down on their exposure to all types of bacteria and germs.

## HOT BUTTON

- Careful food preparation begins with buying food that looks in top form, and washing all fresh produce you bring home.
- Don't forget the importance of keeping hot foods hot and cold foods cold.

# Botulism

Botulism, a life-threatening paralytic illness, is the most lethal form of food poisoning that exists. In the United States, approximately 250 cases of botulism are reported each year.

The illness is transmitted by eating food containing the toxin, and the onset of symptoms usually occurs within 12–36 hours.

There are two particularly difficult aspects of dealing with botulism:

**1.** The microorganism, *Clostridium botulinum,* has the ability to form a spore that is very resistant to heat and chemicals. Because of this resistance, it is more difficult to kill off than other forms of illness-bearing organisms.

**2.** It only takes a taste. One woman tested a bit of her home-canned carrots. Deciding there was something wrong, she threw them out. Within two days she was suffering from botulism. This story is typical of the way botulism works.

The most commonly involved foods are home-canned or commercially canned or processed low-acid vegetables, meats, fish, and poultry that have been insufficiently heated during processing or canning. These include peas, corn, lima beans, green beans, mushrooms, sauces, and soups.

Several conditions are needed for a botulism outbreak:

- the botulinum organism must be in the food.
- the food is being canned or processed in some way; the toxin can form only in the absence of oxygen, so a sealed container such as a can or jar provides ideal conditions.
- inadequate processing or heating lets spores live and toxins form.
- the food is not heated enough before it is eaten to kill the toxin.

You will never get botulism from fresh foods or from acidic food products such as orange juice, pickles, or regular tomatoes (not the low-acid type).

## SYMPTOMS

The toxin affects the central nervous system and interrupts nervous impulses. The illness progresses from difficulty in walking and swallowing and impaired vision and speech to occasional convulsions and ultimately to paralysis of the respiratory muscles, suffocation, and death, all within a few hours or days.

## PREVENTION

Most outbreaks of botulism come from home canning. However, because things very occasionally go wrong with commercial processing, you should know the signs:

- Discard all raw or canned food that shows any sign of spoilage.
- Discard all bulging or swollen cans of food and food from glass jars with bulging lids. (Toxin production creates gases that expand the contents.) If you find them on the store shelves, point them out to the management. Even if you're in a rush, the extra moments it takes to point out bulging cans may save the life of someone who doesn't know the danger signs.
- If you open a can and the contents spurt out explosively, don't eat them.
- *Do not taste* food from swollen containers or food that is foamy or has a bad odor. When in doubt, throw it out.
- A frequent cause of infant botulism is honey, so don't give honey to babies who are less than a year old.
- The organism that causes botulism is found in soil all over the world, so cover open wounds when they may get dirty.

## TAKE CARE WITH HOME CANNING

Prevention of botulism is extremely important. Home canning should follow strict hygienic recommendations to reduce contamination of foods.

- There are no shortcuts to home canning. It takes time, proper equipment, proper processing, and exact information on preparation.
- Contact your County Cooperative Extension Office for information. They can provide you with the latest safety guidelines.
- Bacterial spores in food can be destroyed by high temperatures (212 degrees Fahrenheit), obtained only in the pressure canner. More than six hours is needed to kill the spores at boiling temperature.
- Consider not eating or permitting your child to eat foods that were canned at home unless you did it yourself and know that it was done safely.
- As an extra precaution, boil home-preserved food for 10–20 minutes before serving. This will destroy the toxin.

## TREATMENT

Intravenous or intramuscular administration of antitoxin is the primary treatment. Fluids are administered to prevent dehydration. The treatment can be effective if started early.

# E. Coli

There are many new developments in trying to eradicate E. coli from our food chain:

- A new machine that instantly tests for the presence of E. coli has just been developed.
- Scientists are experimenting with feeding cattle differently to reduce the presence of the bacteria in that part of the food chain.
- A biotech company in Canada has just developed the first drug to treat the condition. In trials the drug has reduced by half the risk of patients who go on to develop hemolytic uremic syndrome (HUS), which is characterized by kidney failure and loss of red blood cells.

Though the indications are that we'll see less and less of E. coli in the future, right now it's still a very present worry, and it's something to take seriously in the way we handle the food we eat.

## ABOUT E. COLI

E. coli is found everywhere in harmless forms, including human intestines. Not until 1982 was E. coli first associated with disease in humans. At that time a rare strain of E. coli (0157:H7) was identified, and it is 0157:H7 that causes people to get sick.

If someone is exposed to 0157:H7, he or she can experience severe damage to the intestines and lose water and salts. Damage to blood vessels and bleeding can occur. This strain of E. coli is particularly damaging to children, the elderly, and the immunosuppressed. In some children it leads to hemolytic uremia syndrome (HUS), and approximagely 5–10 percent of children who become ill progress to this stage.

It's estimated that 20,000 Americans get sick from E. coli poisoning each year and about 200 die. For those who become ill, there is the risk of kidney failure and death.

## HOW IT SPREADS

While undercooked meat is most frequently the way people become infected with E. coli, it can also be present in drinking water (see "Your Water Supply"), and fresh foods that may have been exposed to contaminated water in irrigation or in later washing of the produce. E. coli is also sometimes present in unpasteurized juices.

Ground beef is a particular hazard, so careful cooking is very important. E. coli lives on the exterior of the meat, so when the meat is ground the contamination spreads throughout the food.

And while you'd like to think your expensive steak couldn't possibly have E. coli inside it, you still have to be careful. One thin knife cut is enough to contaminate the meat inside, at which point making certain the steak is cooked well enough becomes of prime importance. (Hamburger needs to reach an internal temperature of at least 160; 145 will be adequate with most other forms of beef.) The safest way to prepare meat is to cook it until the juices run absolutely clear.

## SYMPTOMS

Symptoms vary, depending on the health of the individual, but in general, the person who consumes harmful E. coli will have fever, vomiting, and blood in the stool. If you see anything worrisome, particularly in a young child, call your doctor immediately.

## PREVENTION

- Wash hands frequently, particularly after handling meat.
- Avoid cross-contamination. Don't take burgers out to the grill and bring them back in on the same plate.
- Always clean any surface that has come in contact with raw meat.

- Always cook meat until juices run clear.
- Don't buy unpasteurized juices. Pasteurization kills E. coli.
- Wash lettuce carefully in cold running water.
- Wash fruit, even those you're peeling, in plain cold water.
- Sprouts have been found to carry E. coli. Until you read otherwise, this is a salad extra you ought to forego.
- If you have to send meat back at a restaurant because it is undercooked, request a clean plate, and in the case of a hamburger, a new bun to avoid cross-contamination.

## CONTAMINATED RECREATIONAL WATERS

(Also see "Your Water Supply.")

Occasionally a pool or beach area will be the source of E. coli, generally through contamination by a swimmer. Even in these cases there are a few measures you can take to protect yourself. Ask that the facility:

- Require all children who are not toilet-trained to wear tight-fitting rubber or plastic pants.
- Post signs warning patrons not to swallow the lake water.
- Avoid overcrowding.
- Provide adequate bathrooms.
- Ask that patrons not use the beach water when suffering from stomach ills.

## ONE TOP TIP TO TEACH CHILDREN ABOUT E. COLI

Because children are particularly vulnerable to E. coli, it is very important that their meat be well cooked. Teach your children not to eat meat that is pink inside.

## HOT BUTTON

- Wash all produce thoroughly.
- Be careful not to cross-contaminate plates and utensils when preparing meat.
- Cook all meat until the juices run clear.

# *Listeria*

Until a recent outbreak in the United States called attention to this relatively unusual illness, listeriosis was not much on the minds of the public. However, in 1998–99 100 illnesses, including 21 deaths (15 adults and 6 miscarriages/stillbirths to mothers) in 22 states, grabbed national newspaper headlines. The villain was recognized as *Listeria*, and the source was identified as a food manufacturer of hot dogs and deli meats.

Suddenly it seemed we couldn't send our children to school with a bologna sandwich without placing them at risk for infection.

## ABOUT *LISTERIA*

According to the CDC, an estimated 1100 people in the U.S. report serious illness from listeriosis each year. Of those reporting, approximately 25 percent die as a result of the illness.

*Listeria*, the organism that causes listeriosis, is often found in soil and water as well as in our own gastrointestinal tracts. While a healthy person might suffer flu-like symptoms occasionally, those who are susceptible—the young, the old, pregnant women (who can pass it on to their fetuses), and those with a suppressed immune system—can become seriously ill. Antibiotics are recommended for treatment of the infection, but in some cases diagnosis is made too late. The incubation period for the illness averages three weeks, but it can take as long as 70 days, so it's not always easy to spot.

One reason we see very little of listeriosis is because *Listeria* can easily be killed by pasteurization and cooking.

## SYMPTOMS

The person with listeriosis generally has flu-like symptoms such as fever and chills—sometimes an upset stomach, but not always. If the infection spreads to the nervous system, symptoms include headache, stiff neck, confusion, loss of balance, or convulsions.

## PREVENTION

- If you or a family member falls into the risk group, reheat until steaming hot (internal temperature of 165 for at least one minute) the following types of ready-to-eat foods: hot dogs, luncheon meats, cold cuts, fermented and dry sausage, and other deli-style meat and poultry products.
- If you cannot reheat foods and you or a family member falls into the risk category, don't eat them.
- Don't drink raw, unpasteurized milk or eat foods made from it such as unpasteurized cheese. Also avoid soft cheeses such as feta, Brie, Camembert, blue-veined, or Mexican-style cheese. Hard cheeses, processed cheeses, cream cheese, cottage cheese, and yogurts carry no danger of *Listeria*.
- Watch expiration dates.
- Wash hands with hot, soapy water after handling these foods to prevent contaminating other foods. (Wash for at least 30 seconds.) Wash cutting boards, dishes, and utensils.
- Refrigeration does not kill *Listeria*, so always use hot soapy water to clean up liquid that spills in the refrigerator from luncheon meats and hot dogs.

## ONE TOP TIP TO TEACH CHILDREN ABOUT *LISTERIA*

Precooked luncheon and deli meats are big favorites of children and are usually a reasonable occasional lunch choice. If, however, you have a child with a suppressed immune system, don't let him eat these foods unless you have reheated them.

## HOT BUTTON

- Unless you're in a high-risk category, *Listeria* should be only a passing worry. Do cook hot dogs to an internal temperature of 165, and watch expiration dates of other products of this type.

# "Mad Cow" Disease—Bovine Spongiform Encephalopathy (BSE)

In the late 1980s a unique set of circumstances in Britain contributed to an epidemic of "mad cow" disease that lasted through 1996. The disease began among cattle, and then in 1995 a human variant of the disease was recognized, causing a great deal of alarm. Since that time, thirty-nine Britons have died from Creutzfeldt-Jakob disease (CJD), the human variant, which they apparently caught from eating contaminated beef.

The epidemic in animals began in 1986 when a bizarre brain disease called bovine spongiform encephalopathy (BSE) began killing cattle in Britain. Infected animals developed spongy areas in their brains, suffered personality changes, and began staggering in circles. These symptoms led to the reference of "mad cow" disease. Almost 200,000 cows were eventually diagnosed with the disease, and more than 4 million were destroyed in an effort to stamp out the infection. The cows apparently became ill because of eating the scrap remains of infected cows, a common practice in some places.

At first British officials assured the public that people could not get the disease from eating beef from infected cattle. However, when young people began to develop Creutzfeldt-Jakob disease, a disease found almost exclusively in people over age 50, scientists began to worry. After additional investigation, researchers showed that the brains of infected cows and those of the young people had identical patterns of disease. The human form of mad cow disease was then named "new variant" CJD. (Older victims develop a form called spontaneous CJD.)

## ABOUT "MAD COW" DISEASE

Mad cow disease is a slowly progressing degenerative disease affecting the central nervous system of cows. It eventually kills by eating holes in the brain tissue of cattle.

In people, the new variant of CJD is characterized by fatigue, memory loss, bizarre behavior, muscle weakness, loss of vision, and paralysis. As in bovine spongiform encephalopathy, the brain becomes riddled with holes; in CJD it also becomes covered with a plaque-like substance.

Because the spontaneous CJD progresses slowly, and can incubate for several decades, those affected tend to be elderly. The tip-off to scientists that they were dealing with a previously unknown form of CJD was when young people started dying of it. This discovery led to connecting the human illness with "mad cow" disease.

## TREATMENT

At present there is no treatment to prevent or stall this fatal disease, though doctors in Britain are getting close to a test that will let them look for the prion protein thought to cause the new form of CJD. This will take them closer to treatment and better prevention.

## PREVENTION

Researchers say that the risk of a human variant of mad cow disease breaking out among Americans is small. The government has banned beef from Europe and taken steps to protect domestic herds from consuming feed that may spread the fatal brain disease.

# Salmonella

Anyone who grew up eating raw cookie dough is not going to enjoy this chapter, for salmonella is still alive and well and doing its part to contribute to food poisoning statistics. It is estimated that 3.8 million Americans are sickened by salmonella annually, and it is the most common food-borne illness in the United States.

## ABOUT SALMONELLA

Salmonella includes over a thousand varieties of bacteria (including one that causes typhoid fever). Salmonella is not actually a case of poisoning, since there is no toxin involved, but it is a systemic infection caused by bacteria. Salmonella can be quite severe and even fatal.

Typically the foods involved in salmonella are fresh ones that have been contaminated with the bacteria through unsanitary handling or fouling by animals. The most frequent foods through which people are infected are eggs, cheese, and other dairy products. Other foods that are carriers include poultry, shellfish, and shrimp as well as meats eaten raw or rare. The salmonella that appears in poultry is the number one bacterium in chicken and is very prevalent.

Though it is uncommon, fruits or vegetables can sometimes be contaminated. Reptiles are carriers of salmonella, so families who own a pet iguana, turtles, lizards, or snakes must take particular care.

## SYMPTOMS

Salmonella causes a swelling in the lining of the small intestine. The resulting disease typically lasts up to a week and can be life-threatening for infants, the elderly, or anyone with a weak immune system.

The symptoms can range from mild to severe diarrheal illness. The incubation period is 8–48 hours after exposure, and the acute illness can last for a week or two.

## TREATMENT

Generally salmonella runs its course, and the person gets better. However, fluids are important for the patient, who will generally have lost a lot of fluids and electrolytes (salt and minerals) through diarrhea.

## PREVENTION

- Buy food only from establishments that handle it properly: frozen foods should be solidly frozen, meats and dairy products should be refrigerated, and fruits and vegetables should appear clean and fresh.
- Wash fresh food well.
- Good hand washing is important, particularly after handling eggs and poultry.

- The salmonella in poultry is destroyed through proper cooking. Chicken, duck, goose, turkey should all be cooked to 180 degrees; parts should be cooked to 170. Fortunately people don't like raw chicken, so they are better about cooking it well.
- Don't eat raw oysters or other uncooked shellfish.
- If you own a reptile, wear gloves when handling the animal or cleaning the cage.

## EXTRA CARE REQUIRED WITH EGGS

Egg-associated salmonellosis is an important public health problem in the United States. According to the U.S. Agriculture Department, nearly 900,000 Americans fall ill each year from eggs contaminated with salmonella. In parts of the United States, the CDC estimates that each year 1 in 50 consumers could be exposed to a contaminated egg.

Unfortunately, perfectly normal-looking eggs can have salmonella inside. (Salmonella infects the ovaries of healthy hens and contaminates the eggs before the shells form.) However, if the egg is thoroughly cooked, the organisms will be destroyed and won't make the person sick.

New government-required warning labels are now on egg cartons, but fortunately, the government seems to be making progress on eradication as well. Farmers are beginning to use a spray on chicks that should eventually reduce the rates of salmonella. In the meantime, here's what to do:

- Shop for pasteurized eggs at your grocery store. Pasteurization kills the salmonella, decreasing your family's exposure to the disease. Eventually, pasteurized eggs may totally dominate the market, making our egg supply much safer.
- Keep eggs refrigerated.
- Discard cracked or dirty eggs.

- Wash hands and cooking utensils with soap and water after contact with raw eggs
- Eat eggs promptly after cooking. Don't keep eggs warm for more than two hours.
- Refrigerate unused or leftover egg-containing foods.
- Avoid eating raw eggs (as in homemade ice cream or eggnog). Commercially manufactured ice cream, mayonnaise, cookie dough, and eggnog are made with pasteurized eggs and have not been linked with salmonella infections.
- Avoid restaurant dishes made with raw or undercooked, unpasteurized eggs. Restaurants should use pasteurized eggs in any recipe (Hollandaise sauce? Caesar salad dressing?) that calls for raw eggs.

## TWO TOP TIPS TO TEACH CHILDREN ABOUT SALMONELLA

1. If your children have been cookie-dough eaters, you need to discourage the practice, or let them have a taste of the butter and sugar before the eggs are added.
2. If they come in contact with a turtle that lives at school or an iguana that lives at their friend's house, teach them the importance of careful hand washing.

## HOT BUTTON

- Wash your hands after you've been in contact with raw eggs or chicken.
- Cook eggs and chicken thoroughly.

# Typhoid Fever

Though there are 33 million cases of typhoid throughout the world each year, typhoid is slowly disappearing from the United States because of the prevalence of preventive measures. Compulsory inspection of milk and water supplies, and the pasteurization of milk, has greatly reduced the incidence of the disease. Another important factor has been the typhoid inoculation of people exposed to the disease such as hospital employees and travelers to areas with poor sanitary facilities. Since the early 1960s the U.S. has reported an annual rate of fewer than 1000 cases per year of typhoid fever, more than half of them contracted by Americans traveling in foreign countries. Infected food handlers are to blame for a good number of the remaining cases.

Typhoid is among the diseases that you can catch from an asymptomatic carrier as well as someone who is sick. The best known individual carrier who lacked symptoms was "Typhoid Mary," a cook named Mary Mallon who spread the disease to hundreds in New York City in the early 1900s before the source of the epidemic was discovered.

## ABOUT TYPHOID FEVER

Typhoid fever is an acute infectious disease caused by the typhoid bacillus *Salmonella typhi*. It is transmitted by milk, water, or solid food contaminated by the feces of typhoid victims or of carriers. It can also be found in fish and shellfish taken from polluted water.

## SYMPTOMS

Typhoid fever has an incubation period of 5–21 days. The symptoms may not be alarming at first, but typhoid will eventually present itself as severe abdominal pain, diarrhea that can be bloody, high fever, intense headache, and a splotchy rash.

Typhoid fever is treatable with antibiotics, but some strains are showing an increased resistance to drugs. Prevention is a better plan of attack against this disease.

## PREVENTION

- Eating in decent restaurants where food handlers maintain proper hygiene is your best protection against the slight risk of encountering a carrier in the United States.
- If you are traveling to countries where the sanitation is questionable, get vaccinated for typhoid fever. It isn't required for entrance to many countries, but why take the risk?
- If there is a natural disaster in an otherwise safe community, a typhoid vaccination might be recommended. If so, have your family inoculated.

## HOT BUTTON

- Get vaccinated if you're traveling to countries where a low level of cleanliness might lead to the spread of this disease.

# The Safety of the Food You Buy

When it comes to shopping for food, most of us look carefully to pick out the most beautiful red tomatoes, the freshest lettuce and worm-free apples. But when food scientists develop methods like genetically altered foods and irradiation to deliver to the marketplace the most attractive, bacteria-free food they can, we pause before buying.

Here's what you should know about some of these methods:

## GENETICALLY ALTERED FOODS

Scientists use two methods to alter foods genetically. The first is the traditional method, called hybridization, which has been done for years. In hybridization, plants with desirable traits are crossed to form offspring with the best traits from both parent plants.

The second and newer method involves transgenic alteration. It involves taking genes from one source and implanting them in another. By using this method, food scientists hope to one day develop broccoli with added nutrients, tomatoes with top-notch taste, low-lactose milk, and sunflower oil with less saturated fat. One day, food altered genetically might also deliver specifically tailored combinations of vitamins and possibly even foods that could serve to prevent or treat ailments.

Thus far, however, most genetically modified foods aren't engineered to boost nutritional content. They are supposed to boost agricultural yields by increasing resistance to insects or to weed killers, a boon to farmers who are looking for ways to grow healthier crops more rapidly.

While there is no proof that bioengineered food poses any health risks, and advocates point out that in addition to creating better foods, insect-resistant plants will reduce the need for pesticides, there are still many unresolved issues.

Certainly, one of the first issues concerns the testing necessary for the products to be approved by the government. To date, there are no specific scientific standards for proving the environmental safety of a plant, nor is there a specific review process for genetically modified foods. However, this issue and the review process are currently being studied.

Labeling is another concern. In the United States, labels identifying genetically modified foods aren't required, and labeling in Europe, where the issue of genetic modification is far more heated, has just recently been mandated. However, the new guidelines ran into trouble almost immediately. Additives and flavorings were initially exempt from being counted, so a food laden with additional additives could still claim to be "GM free"; this regulation is in the process of being changed. There is also ongoing discussion about how "GM free" something has to be to claim that status. The European Union, which is empowered to provide this type of legislation for its fifteen member countries, is currently considering stipulating that products don't require labeling if each of the ingredients contains 1 percent bioengineered material or less. Consumer groups are arguing for a limit of one-tenth of that.

Unpredictable allergic reaction is another concern, though foods containing any substance known to cause allergies (such as nuts or any oil from nuts) is to be labeled as such.

In the United States, we've already been eating from a food web that contains genetically modified foods. About 55 percent of soybeans and 30 percent of corn are modified. What's different about the new products that are being developed is that for the first time the plants are capable of reproducing, and this has caused great concern among ecologists. If the transgene from a genetically modified plant crosses into the wild population, then a new SuperWeed may be created. Some genetic alterations may actually stunt the growth of other types of plants with which it can be cross-pollinated.

The American public finally woke up to the alarm being expressed by Europeans when it was discovered that genetically altered corn carries a toxin that, when spread to the common milkweed plant that is a frequent intruder in cornfields, kills monarch butterflies, which feed on milkweed. In a final twist of irony, the genetically altered plants may, in some cases, endanger varieties of plants that scientists still rely on to provide the raw material for the genetic alterations.

While improved biotechnology—creating a crop that remedies the bug problem, but doesn't affect the plants' pollen, for example—may ultimately be an answer, there is great concern among ecologists that the U.S. government has given approval to grow these genetically changed plants without yet having seen the results of long-term studies of their effects on the environment. The tremendous profit potential for industry, as well as a very real pressure for increased food production, has made it tempting to adopt a short-term view of the risks and benefits of putting genetically modified crops on the fast track.

Despite all these issues, many scientists still argue that transgenic alteration of plants is actually safer than hybridization (something that's taken place for so long, no one has ever thought to question it), because working with genetic material is more precise than cross-breeding plant families. A valid point made by the naysayers is that continued testing is important to any type of experimentation done with foods.

I urge you to keep up-to-date on this issue, as it's guaranteed to be a frequent news story in the coming years.

## IRRADIATION

By exposing foods to ionized radiation, food scientists have discovered an effective way to destroy many of the pathogens that have been causing food poisoning.

As a technology, it's been around for forty years, and it's likely that it will be used more and more as a method of keeping our food safe. O. Sue Snider, Ph.D., a food and nutrition specialist at the University of Delaware, says: "You get a minimal amount of change in the food, no more than the nutrient destruction in cooking the food. The benefit is the food you're eating is safe."

Lester M. Crowford, D.V.M., Ph.D., Director of the Georgetown Center for Food and Nutrition Policy in Washington, D.C., is quoted in a scientific report on the safety of irradiation of food as saying: "It is safer to irradiate the food than to not irradiate it . . ."

## PESTICIDES

Part of eating worm-free apples and beating the bugs to the spinach leaves must be attributed to the fact that farmers use pesticides. For most of us, the level permitted by the federal government is safe enough that it won't do us noticeable harm, but in some cases, the levels of toxicity on fruits and vegetables is higher than what we would want our children to consume. Children tend to eat more produce per pound of body weight than adults, and they are more sensitive to some pesticides.

Some protection lies in eating organic foods, which are not exposed to chemical pesticides. However, nutritionists are quick to point out that organic foods should not be considered danger-free. As we return to the "natural" methods, we also return to the potential pathogens that the chemicals have been created to eradicate. Ingesting bacterial microbes that may make us sick is a possibility when eating organic food. For some families, the fact that prices are higher for organic foods will also be a factor.

## THE SOLUTION LIES IN BALANCE

Scientists who specialize in food safety say that "balance" and safe preparation are key.

- Serve a wide variety of fresh food. This is particularly helpful for children. If people eat a range of fresh foods, it minimizes their exposure to any one type of chemical.
- Wash all fresh food well in cold running water. Peel as needed. Don't use soap in the washing process. Fresh produce is very porous, the detergent will be absorbed, and the effects of detergent in the body are untested.
- Be aware of how food is regulated in your state and locality. If you think the food you're purchasing doesn't look fresh, find out to whom you can complain.

## ONE TOP TIP TO TEACH YOUR CHILDREN ABOUT FOOD SAFETY

Encourage your children to eat a wide variety of foods to minimize their exposure to any one potentially dangerous chemical.

## HOT BUTTON

- Wash fresh foods carefully in cold water to reduce the risk from pesticides.
- Stay abreast of what is happening in food development. To let the FDA know you're concerned, write to the FDA Commissioner, HF-2, 5600 Fishers Lane, Rockville, MD 20857.

# Chapter 10

# Dangerous Encounters with Animals and Insects

## Introduction

B ees kill about fifty Americans a year, domestic dogs another twenty, rattlesnakes a dozen. Roughly a hundred people in the United States die each year when their cars meet deer on roads and highways.

Human encounters with wild animals are part of a growing phenomenon occurring in all parts of the nation and involve animals as diverse as mountain lions, bears, alligators, and snakes. Wildlife experts believe there are many reasons why wild animal attacks are seemingly on the rise, but two certainly explain many of them—proximity and provocation.

With hunting on the decline, species such as deer are growing in population, and with the success of wildlife conservation programs, we're seeing an increase in animals just at the time when more people are moving into once-remote areas. As a result, humans and potentially dangerous wildlife are seeing more of each other. In Florida, the population increases by 1000 people each day, and some of those people are moving into homes on land that formerly belonged to alligators; in mountain states, joggers and cougars are traveling some of the same paths. Subdivisions,

summer homes, heavily trafficked parks, diverse and intense outdoor recreation all put people and animals into close contact.
This contact also causes animals to lose their innate fear of humans. The desensitization of animals is one of the most dangerous developments of all.

Proximity and provocation are also part of the problem in our
national parks, where people think they are visiting an environment that is as controlled as Disney World. The vast majority of
injuries that occur in the parks happen because people forget
that they are in the wild. Though bison are never thought of as
threatening to humans, a good number of people have been
charged and gored by these 1800-pound beasts when people
have come close to take a picture or have taunted or tormented
the animals from close range. In a nature park in the South, a father started to lift his child into a pen with alligators in order to
take a picture of the child with the alligator. Only the keeper's
quick maneuver to get the child back out again kept her from becoming the reptile's lunch.

A recent article in *The New York Times* put it into perspective:
The beloved dolphin, long felt to be as friendly to man as its
seemingly "smiling" countenance implies, has been shown to
have a dark side; dolphins practice both infanticide and the
bludgeoning of porpoises, for no discernible reason (dolphins
don't eat what they kill in these instances). This is a "friendly"
mammal around which entire recreational industries have been
built, including dolphin performances at aquariums and boating
expeditions to observe them, not to mention the businesses devoted to helping people swim with dolphins in both captivity
and the wild. While human injuries have thus far been low (less
than 1 in 10,000), experts who study the matter say it's only a matter of time until there's a tragic accident.

Disease, too, often spreads from animals to people. As we find
ourselves living side by side with wild animals and insects, science has made us aware that some of the sicknesses that befall
us stem from this proximity. The final chapters in this section ad-

dress a few of the animal- and insect-borne illnesses that cause worry.

Whether it's as tiny as a bee or as big as a bear, that insect, reptile, or animal has its own set of likes and dislikes. The better we are at learning what those preferences are and respecting them, the more likely we are to emerge from any encounter unscathed.

# Alligators

The larger varieties of both alligators and crocodiles have the power to kill swiftly and without warning. If you're in America, you're far more likely to encounter the American alligator. If traveling outside the country (in the Nile region and countries such as Australia—remember *Crocodile Dundee?*), you'll need to watch out for the crocodile. Both are reptiles and members of the order Crocodylia. Though each has distinguishing physical characteristics, being grabbed by either one would feel about the same.

In Florida, the state with the highest alligator population in the United States, the once-endangered reptile has bounced back from near extinction. As the state's burgeoning human population encroaches on the alligator's habitat, human–alligator contact has increased. There have been 248 alligator attacks on humans since 1948, when the count began; half of them involved children; nine were fatal. What's worrisome is that four of the fatal attacks have occurred in the last five years.

Much of the problem stems from the increase in familiarity. Generally, alligators are eager to get away from humans, but as the species has become more accustomed to people, their fear has begun to subside.

"The situation is made even worse when people feed the alligators," says a spokesperson with the Florida Game and Freshwater Fish Commission. "They visit a lake regularly, begin to call the alligator who lives there 'Old Joe,' and they give him scraps from their picnic. The alligators begin to associate people with food, and the next thing you know, Old Joe decides a little boy playing in the water is his next meal."

## ABOUT ALLIGATORS AND CROCODILES

The order of Crocodylia should be thought of as the order of the Great Survivors. For over 70 million years the crocodile has remained virtually unchanged; they are the only great reptile predator to have outlived the dinosaurs. Some say they have been on the earth for 200 million years.

In the late 1770s naturalist William Bartram described the St. Johns River in Florida as having alligators "in such incredible numbers and so close together from shore to shore that it would have been easy to have walked across on their heads had the animals been harmless."

As civilization moved in and people destroyed their habitats by draining swamps and killing off the reptiles to make shoes and purses, the Florida alligator population decreased and was nearly wiped out. When the reduction in numbers became obvious, hunting was restricted, but illegal poaching continued through the 1960s, when effective legislation was finally passed. Now the American alligator is protected by law. It can be commercially farmed, but it can only be killed by special permit to get rid of "nuisance alligators." This has led to the resurgence of the alligator.

Today the American alligator is found in swamps and sluggish streams from North Carolina to Florida and along the Gulf Coast. Though these alligators at one time commonly grew to 18 feet in length, the longer reptiles are now very rare. The most commonly sighted ones today are more likely to be about ten feet long. Alligators spend their days floating just below the surface of the water or resting on the bank; they spend nights hunting on the bank and in the water. They are most active during the spring mating season, which lasts until June. Young alligators feed on water insects, crustaceans, frogs, and fish. As they grow, they catch proportionately larger animals. Alligators occasionally catch and kill deer or cows that come to drink, but most attacks on humans are in self-defense, or because they've become too accustomed to living among two-legged beasts.

Crocodiles are distinguished from alligators by the presence of a long lower fourth tooth that protrudes on the side of the head when the mouth is closed. The snouts of most crocodiles are narrower than those of alligators.

In southern Florida, the North American Saltwater Crocodile is making a reappearance after a quick brush with extinction. Like the alligator, the species once swarmed around the southern peninsula of Florida, but it, too, was almost wiped out by developers and poachers. By the 1970s only 200–300 survived. Today conservationists have helped bring the numbers back to apoximately 600 in the saltwater areas around South Florida. As a species, they are shy and timid and up until recently very rare.

Though pets have frequently become prey to these crocodiles, there has not yet been an attack on a human in the United States However, as crocodiles continue to move into yards and golf courses in the area, an unfortunate encounter with a human seems inevitable.

All species play a role in the natural order of things. One of the most important services performed by these reptiles—beyond their role as predators—is the creation of mud holes. To stay cool, they use their bodies to make small craters in the ground in marshland areas. Water then collects in these gator holes, and during a dry spell, these holes may hold the only water in the area for crayfish, turtles, frogs, fish, and insects. Otters, raccoons, great blue herons, and water snakes are able to survive because of the continued existence of the creatures who created the water hole.

## DON'T FEED THE ALLIGATORS!

Feeding these reptiles is felt to be the primary reason for the increase in attacks. When fed, they overcome their natural shyness and become accustomed or attracted to humans. Wildlife experts are perturbed by the public's refusal to heed these warnings.

- If you see someone feeding alligators, tell them it can lead to an attack. (If you're in Florida, you can tell them it's a violation of state law.)
- Don't throw fish scraps into the water or leave them on shore—you're unintentionally feeding alligators. Use designated garbage areas.

## TO REDUCE THE LIKELIHOOD OF ATTACK

- When walking, avoid areas with thick vegetation along shorelines; these areas provide good natural habitat for large alligators.
- If you are near a river or its bank, be extremely cautious. Alligators are capable of gliding toward you silently, showing only their eyes above water. They can surge quickly out of the water if they want to attack.
- Don't swim outside posted swimming areas or in waters that might contain large alligators. In Florida there don't tend to be warning signs about alligators because nearly every body of water in Florida has the big reptiles. In other words, if it isn't marked for swimming, assume the area belongs to an alligator.
- Swim with a partner at all times.
- Don't swim at night or dusk when alligators most actively feed.
- Don't allow pets to swim near waters known to contain large alligators. Dogs suffer more attacks than humans, probably because they resemble natural prey.

- If an alligator has wandered onto land (your driveway? the path by your hotel?), leave it alone. The alligator will generally retreat to more preferred habitats away from people.
- If you encounter an alligator that poses a threat:

  ◆ Don't get near the alligator. While they are not fast enough to chase you down, they are still quite agile and very strong. Most land attacks occur when they are able to corner a pet against a fence.
  ◆ Don't harass it. Your potential for being bitten or injured by a thrashing alligator are high.

- If you're concerned about a particular alligator, call the game and wildlife commission in your area.

## IF AN ATTACK OCCURS:

- Remain as calm as you can. Use anything available—a knife or your fingers—to poke at their eyes or nostrils while making as much noise as possible.
- Crocodiles get tired when the victim keeps fighting. Shouting and hitting may save you.

## TWO TOP TIPS TO TEACH CHILDREN ABOUT ALLIGATORS

1. "Never smile at a crocodile" goes for alligators, too. Teach your children to get an adult if they find an alligator in their pathway.
2. Teach children to swim only in designated swimming areas.

## HOT BUTTON

- Never feed an alligator, and try to prevent others from doing so.
- If an alligator is hanging around your house or yard and doesn't seem to be returning to his natural habitat, call the game and wildlife commission or the animal control agency.
- If attacked by an alligator, fight back.

# Bats

Bats are the only mammal capable of sustained flight, and they are valuable to us ecologically and economically. Some species cross-pollinate plants, and almost all bats work as "bug catchers of the night." A single bat can devour up to 600 mosquitoes in an hour, and for that alone we should be extremely grateful.

Unfortunately, they also carry rabies. Both people and animals can get rabies from contact with a rabid bat, through a bite, a scratch, or saliva contact to your eyes, nose, mouth, or an open wound. In some parts of the nation, particularly western Washington, as many as one in ten bats carries rabies. However, nationally rabies-carrying bats comprise less than 1 percent of the bat population.

What's frightening is that from 1990–98, 27 people nationally died of rabies, and 20 of those deaths were attributed to bats. Many of the victims had no recollection of having come into contact with a bat, meaning that in many cases diagnosis of rabies comes too late to be of help. (Treatments need to be under way before symptoms occur.) The process of diagnosing is further complicated by the fact that the incubation for rabies can be weeks or even months. In addition, the teeth and claws of the bat are often so tiny and so exceedingly sharp that they can actually puncture a person's skin without causing pain.

## ABOUT BATS

Bats can range in size from the Kitti's hog-nosed bat, which weighs less than a penny, to the fruit bat, whose wingspan can reach six feet. They prey on migrating moths, bloodsucking mosquitoes, and crop-eating pests. Many bats will eat nearly their body weight in insects before dawn. Exceptional fliers, they are able to fly at low speeds with better maneuverability than most birds.

Bats navigate by echolocation. They make high-pitched sounds that then bounce off objects and back to the bats, telling them where and how big the object is. Despite their very sophisticated navigation system, and contrary to popular opinion, bats aren't blind. Most have excellent vision. The California leaf-nosed bat can see a caterpillar the size of a rice grain by starlight.

Are there really vampire bats? Yes, but they rarely attack humans. They live mostly in the American tropics. They bite their prey—generally an animal—to wound, not to kill, and then use their tongue to lick the blood from the oozing laceration.

The anticlotting enzyme in vampire bats may prove useful in medicine. Research scientists are trying to isolate the chemical that could help in dissolving blood clots and thus aid in the prevention of heart attacks and strokes.

The silver-haired/eastern pipistrelle bat is the species of bat that most frequently transmits rabies to humans. Although it is not a particularly common type of bat, it seems to carry an extremely virulent strain of rabies and has developed a special talent for infecting through minute, shallow wounds. Because the bat's teeth are so small, the bite is almost impossible to detect. People frequently don't realize they've been bitten, making them unaware that they need to seek medical attention.

Bats can be found in all fifty states, and they will always be around us. However, there are ways to minimize the possibility of being exposed to a disease-carrying bat.

## BATPROOF YOUR HOME

- Put screens on doors, windows, and fireplaces. Keep the fireplace or woodstove damper closed.
- Bats can pass through crevices as small as a pencil. Places that can allow bats entry should be caulked or covered with bird netting, fly screening, sheet metal, or wood. Check for openings around your chimney, beneath fascia board or under siding. Check for loose shingles and open up the eaves under your roof. Bats prefer to be in a place that is dark and confined, so if they feel exposed in a specific area, they are less likely to roost. In addition, window shutters should be installed an inch or more from the wall to allow more light and ventilation behind them.
- The best time to bat-proof is late fall through winter when bats are hibernating or at night when they are out.
- If a colony of bats has already settled in your attic, call a specialist. The "home remedies"—lights and moth balls—won't do the trick. A professional will know an effective, humane way to eliminate the bats.

## IF A BAT FLIES INTO YOUR HOME

- If a bat comes into your house, it should be captured and tested for rabies. Try to isolate the bat by closing it into a room (close the closet doors, too). Don't turn on the lights or it will hide. Unless the bat can be captured and tests negative for rabies, you and anyone else in the household should almost certainly begin treatment. Call your local health authority for advice.

## IF YOU ENCOUNTER A BAT OUTSIDE YOUR HOME

- Avoid contact with a sick or dead bat on the ground. If it's behaving oddly, stay away (keep pets away, too), and call animal control services.

- Don't pick up a bat in your yard. You don't even want to brush your hand against it because rabies can be transmitted even after the bat is dead.
- As soon as a grounded bat is found, it should be isolated to prevent further contact with people and animals. If you can, cover it with a pail or coffee can and place a heavy object on top of the container to secure it. Call your local health authority and arrange for it to be tested.
- If your pet could have been in contact with the bat, call your vet.

## TREATMENT

Exposure to rabies is now treated by a series of five injections that are usually given in a muscle, not the stomach as was formerly done. Treatment should be considered if:

- The bat is found to be rabid.
- The bat is not available for testing or the tests were inconclusive.
- The bat is in a bedroom where someone was sleeping.

If there was any possibility that a bat made contact with an unattended young child, a sleeping individual, a person who had been drinking or was on drugs, or a person with sensory or medical impairment, then the bat should be tested.

For more information, see "Rabies."

## TWO TOP TIPS TO TEACH CHILDREN ABOUT BATS

1. Bats can be extremely dangerous, so instill in your child the importance of staying away from them.
2. If a child sees a bat in the house or has any reason to feel

that contact was made with the bat, he or she should tell an adult right away.

## HOT BUTTON

- If you see a bat, leave it alone. Don't swing or throw anything at the bat. Call pest control or animal control services.
- Most bats will find their way out of your home. Leave one opening—door or window—and they'll navigate out through it.
- If there was any chance of contact, have the victim start the series of shots.

# Bears

Statistically, you're far more likely to be hurt in a car accident on the way to a national park, or struck by lightning once there, than you are to be attacked by a bear. However, because bear attacks can and do occur (headlines this year told of an Alaskan resident who was killed while hiking near his home), it's important to know how to handle yourself while hiking. Proper behavior while out on the trail greatly decreases the odds of a bear attack.

In general, bears are poor hosts and hostesses when they don't know you're coming. If you notify them of your arrival by making noise as you hike, they usually scamper away. That's exactly what you want from animals that can weigh 600–700 pounds, reach ten feet up in the air, have razor-sharp claws, and sprint 35–40 miles per hour for a short distance—faster than a racehorse, and twice as fast as the speediest human.

According to bear expert Stephen Herrero, professor of Environmental Design at the University of Calgary, Alberta, and author of *Bear Attacks: Their Causes and Avoidance*, every bear encounter is different, and while some general rules can be provided, avoidance is the best policy. If you're actually in an attack situation, there is no sure prediction of what will happen.

Bears, too, are changing. Years ago, human presence would almost always drive bears away; today wildlife experts are reporting that at times bears will actually stalk to kill. While these occasions are still rare, it means that if you're planning to visit bear country, you need to be aware.

## GET TO KNOW YOUR BEARS

If you're going on a hiking expedition, chances are you've done a lot of research, investigating what gear you need, how you'll get to the trails, and what you'll see along the way. This is all well and good, but you also need to do some research into what to expect from the wildlife you may encounter.

- Find out what kind of bears you might see where you're hiking. Anyone knowledgeable about the area can fill you in on what type of bear behavior to expect and where to be particularly careful. For example, black bears (common in the northern United States and Canada) climb trees; grizzlies (American northwest, Alaska, and western Canada) are less likely to do so.
- Black and brown bears are true hibernators, going without food or elimination of metabolic wastes for three to five months. Because of this, hikers in most areas can actually breathe easier in the winter months, knowing that the likelihood of meeting a bear is reduced. If you're hiking in territory where there are polar bears, they live on a different schedule. Though they don't actually hibernate, they do go without food in the summer, making this a safer time for hikers.
- Some bears wander at night; others move around during the daytime. As a result, your highest "on the trail" bear population will be at dawn and dusk, when both "night"

bears and "day" bears may be prowling around. Try to stay off the trails at these times.

- Stay away from stream bottoms, avalanche chutes, late-summer berry patches, and dense edge cover where bears are more likely to be.
- Stay away from any type of carcass. A bear feeding on a carcass spells big trouble for you.

## PACK WISELY AND THINK AHEAD

For any hiking trip into bear country (a national park or open wilderness), take along the following anti-bear devices:

- Pack a noisemaker; many hikers use a can filled with nuts and bolts because the metal on metal sound is distinctly human. A bell or tin can full of pebbles also work. Professionals don't like what they call "yum yum bells," because they're more annoying and actually less effective than the human voice or banging on something (the sound of the bells doesn't travel as well). What's more, the constant sound of a bell that you actually wear may hinder your ability to hear an animal moving through the underbrush.
- Put pencil flares in an easily accessible pocket of your pack; a flash of light may deter a bear, giving you time to retreat.
- Arm yourself with pepper spray in a belt holster. Created specifically as a bear deterrent, this type of pepper spray uses capsicum, the spicy-hot component found in peppers. The best styles of spray emit an atomized fog and are clearly labeled "bear deterrent." This spray does not deter all bears, and its effectiveness is sometimes limited by thick brush, wind, and rain, but it's one more bit of ammo in your belt. If you're traveling by commercial aircraft to the area where you'll be hiking, you won't be able to carry pepper spray on the plane, even if it's packed in your luggage. Buy

it near where you are going or mail it to yourself "general delivery" in the town near where your hike begins.

*Practice using the spray a time or two,* unfastening the safety cap and giving a quick spray. If you wear contacts, take them out before experimenting. Pepper spray should not be used as a substitute for standard safety procedures. Pepper spray is effective at times, but since distance, wind, rainy weather, and product shelf life can all affect its ability to deter a bear, don't let it make you overly cavalier about hiking in bear country.

- Pack clothing that is 100 percent clean and free of food smells. Your sleeping bag and backpack should also be totally clean. As you travel, anything that gets a food scent on it will have to be stored in the "bear bag" overnight.
- Pack foods like pastas and grains that won't give off an odor that will attract bears.

## TRAIL PREP

- Plan to go with at least one other person. Hiking alone in bear country isn't advisable.
- Learn how—or take along someone who already knows how—to pack and hoist a "bear bag" off the ground. Food items need to be double or triple-bagged in Zip-loc plastic bags, put in a large trash bag or a cloth sack of that type, and tied with a nylon cord and hoisted at least 12 feet into the air (usually between two trees and 8 feet or more away from the trunks of the trees). Personal-care items like soap, sunscreen, and toothpaste should go in the bear bag as well; they, too, emit an odor that is enticing to bears.
- If you're hiking in an area with no trees, or if it's simply more convenient, you can take along bear-proof containers to store food, supplies, and anything that has an odor to it.
- Learn the basics about making camp in bear country—camp away from bear trails, keep no food in the tent, cook

downwind of the tent, remember to hang the bear bag, and get rid of garbage (burn it or pack it into your "bear bag" or bear-proof container).

## NEVER SCARE A BEAR

Silence on the trail is a bad thing. Several long-distance runners have been mauled on hiking trails, almost surely because they were running silently and surprised the bear. Many bear confrontations occur along good fishing streams (for bears as well as humans), where the rushing water masks the noise of approaching hikers.

If given enough warning, bears will react to you the way they react to most humans—they'll go away. Your job is to look, act, sound, and smell human.

- Two or more hikers maintaining a running dialogue in a conversational tone will avoid up-close encounters.
- If you see fresh bear scat, or if you're traveling in bear country in areas where you have limited vision (around blind curves, hiking through terrain or vegetation that limits your vision), you can also clap, sing, talk loudly, or make metallic noise by clanging cups, spoons, or using your noise-maker.

## IF YOU SEE A BEAR, YOU NEED TO START MAKING CHOICES, THE FIRST ONE BEING INVIOLATE

- **Don't Run.** With the ability to run 40 miles per hour, the bear can outrun you, so don't even try that method.
- Try to retreat. If you're intent on proceeding, retreat for five to ten minutes and then return, making noise. If the bear still remains, go back and notify officials if any are nearby. Failing to go away isn't natural behavior for a bear.

- Coming upon a mother bear with her cubs is particularly dangerous. If you have an opportunity to retreat, do so. Don't spend even a moment looking at those cute cubs. Get out before the mother sees you.
- If the bear notices you during the retreat, drop a nonfood item (water bottle, camera, bandana) to distract her. It may give you an extra few minutes to get away.
- If you encounter each other unexpectedly, stop, stay calm and quiet. Break eye contact—as with a dog, a bear interprets a direct stare as a sign of aggression. Back away slowly, apologizing in a quiet, monotone voice (you don't exactly have to say you're sorry, but you ought to convey that idea—and actually you probably would be). You're trying to communicate the bear's dominance and your submissiveness and lack of threat to this animal.
- Don't try climbing a tree. The bear may follow.
- Get your pepper spray ready.

## IF THE BEAR CHARGES YOU

- At this point you're better off standing your ground and using your pepper spray if you have it. Aim your spray at his face or spray a cloud that the bear has to run through to get to you.
- If you have no pepper spray, or if the wind seems to be blowing back to you, which will render the spray ineffective on the bear and unpleasant for you, throw rocks or anything you can. You may be able to scare him away. The bear is usually bluffing in a first charge, and he'll stop short and walk away. If you move suddenly, it may trigger an attack.

## IF HE DOESN'T GO AWAY, FIGHT
## AS LONG AS POSSIBLE

- Toss things (rocks, your noisemaker) at the bear, yell, and do anything you can to resist becoming the bear's next meal. If you've got a stick or anything to swing at the bear, aim at the nose—the most sensitive part of his anatomy. One woman rescued her husband from a mauling by swinging binoculars at the bear and clipping him hard on the nose. It scared him away.
- If you seem to have no alternative, play dead. You are very likely to be hurt at this point, and your strategy needs to minimize the harm that can be done to you. (If you lie down before you're forced to, the bear will almost certainly approach and take a few swipes.)
- While the fetal position has long been believed to be the safest position under these circumstances, bear expert Herrero has come to believe that lying flat facedown is safer. If you were hiking when the encounter occurred, then you are likely still wearing your pack, which will provide a layer of protection. If the bear claws you to flip you over, you can continue the flip and try to lie flat again.
- Try to remain calm during the attack—as painful as it is, doing so may save your life.

## IF YOU LIVE IN BEAR COUNTRY

- Avoid providing any type of food "rewards" that might attract bears to your property. Take down bird feeders in early April, and don't feed pets outside.
- Store your garbage in bear-proof containers.

## TWO TOP TIPS TO TEACH CHILDREN ABOUT BEARS

1. Children who are accompanying you on a hiking trip should be carefully instructed to stay right with you at all times.
2. Kids will be delighted to partake in the "noisemaking" aspect of the hike. Discourage screaming or overly wild behavior, but explain to them that the intent is to let the bears know you're coming. You might even suggest that they simply say (over and over): "Hello, Mr. Bear. We're coming! Hello, Mr. Bear. We're coming!"

## HOT BUTTON

- Never hike alone in bear country.
- Make plenty of noise as you go. Bears don't like surprises— and neither will you.
- If you encounter a bear, act submissive and try to retreat quietly. Don't run.
- Practice what you would do in a bear attack. Unless you've practiced playing dead or backing away, or even looking ahead and staying alert, it will be hard to remember what to do.

# Cockroaches, Mice, and Rats

Cockroaches, mice, and rats are, unfortunately, not an infrequent problem in homes and apartments. While we often find ourselves coexisting with them, it doesn't mean we like it. Here's what you should know about ridding your home environment of these pests. If you think you have an easy task, you don't.

## THE MIGHTY COCKROACH

Cockroaches have been on this earth for longer than you can imagine—before the dinosaurs and before the crocodiles (which predated the dinosaurs); they existed long before there were any mammals at all. They are fast (they can run 50 body lengths per second or about three miles per hour), they can leap hurdles, and if they need to, they can actually get up on their hind legs and run just like we do. They are very versatile and breed quickly, which is why they seem to outlast just about anything. They've even survived nuclear testing and trips into outer space.

While their staying power may be admirable, they aren't much fun to have around. You'd likely lose your appetite if you went to the kitchen at night and turned on the light, only to be greeted by the sight of scurrying bugs.

Scientists have determined that cockroaches track germs around our eating surfaces and that the dust left from decaying cockroaches causes asthma.

Exterminators are the first to admit that cockroaches are their toughest enemy. Partly because cockroaches are highly resistant to many insecticides, exterminators today use organic sprays containing organonphosphates, carbamates, and pyrethroids, which attack the cockroaches' nervous systems. If poison is necessary, hydramethylnon, a gradual metabolic poison, is now the preferred method.

To combat cockroaches, you'll need to work on cleaning out the places where they live and then trying to trap them:

- If you live in an apartment complex, ask the building management to hire a pest control company to treat all the infested units at one time. Fighting the problem in your apartment will be impossible if they are elsewhere in the building.
- Keep the kitchen clean and remove garbage regularly.

- Make sure plumbing leaks and other sources of moisture are repaired or eliminated.
- Pick up papers, boxes, and other clutter that give cockroaches places to hide.
- Make sure that cracks and spaces in walls, around pipes, and near wiring are sealed.
- When it comes to home remedies, boric acid and sticky traps (Roach Motels) may be helpful. Place traps throughout your home, especially in the kitchen and in the bathroom. (Place at least one trap under each sink.) Place traps tight against the walls so the roaches can't go behind them.
- To avoid taking cockroaches with you when you move, pack your belongings during the day and then store them overnight outside the apartment in a cockroach-free environment. If that isn't possible, place boxes off the floor and away from walls on tables and chairs.
- Watch for cockroaches when boxes are being unpacked. If you spy stowaway roaches, try to kill them before they multiply.

While odds are that roaches will survive for all time, scientists are working on inventions that might help control their numbers and locations. It would be great if humans didn't actually have to live with them.

One day our kitchen cabinets might feature air-puffing devices. Scientists at Alabama Agricultural Experiment Station in Auburn, Alabama, are working on a system that plays on the cockroaches' dislike of moving air. After learning that a steady puff of air keeps cockroaches moving, the inventors began creating a device to fit into the back of a cabinet or around the refrigerator that would serve as an environmentally friendly way of keeping cockroaches away from their favorite habitats.

## RODENTS

Most of us respond with more than a mild "EEEK" when we find a mouse or a rat in our household.

One Connecticut family first learned they were sharing their home with the Martha Stewart of rats when a small marzipan snowman disappeared from their holiday display. The still-intact snowman was later found "decorating" the space under the dishwasher where a rat was living. Despite the whimsical idea that the rat had actually decorated his living space, the family felt compelled to call an exterminator.

Human beings are the best things that ever happened to mice and rats. In addition to providing handy holiday decorations for vermin households, people build nice, warm, dry places to live that offer mice and rats the perfect option when it's time to move somewhere warm for the winter.

One of the most common types of mice people find in their homes is the house mouse. It's small, about three inches long, grayish brown, and the most prevalent mouse species in North America. The species is very prolific; the female usually has five to ten litters per year, and each litter can number in the teens.

One of the most common ailments mice and rats can spread is salmonellosis, or more simply, food contamination. Salmonella bacteria are spread through mice feces, but the excrement doesn't have to come in direct contact with the food to spread the disease. Containers, wrappers, and other material on the shelves and countertops where mice run can also transfer the bacteria from feces to food.

A mouse or rat bite can transmit Haverhill fever, which can cause fever, chills, vomiting, headache, or muscle and joint pain. Other less common but serious health problems can stem from rat and mouse infestation, including hantavirus (see Hantavirus). Occasionally, there have been rodent-caused cases of bubonic plague.

Mice and rats also present a safety hazard when they gnaw through electrical wiring.

Here are some steps to take to reduce the likelihood of having rodents in your home:

- If you buy bulk foods, keep them in plastic or ceramic containers with lids. If you live in the country, keep all food in containers or in the refrigerator or freezer. Cooking utensils—plates and forks, knives, and spoons—should be kept in containers as well.
- Check your home for openings in screen doors, where pipes come in and out of the house, and vents. Mice and rats are climbers so the opening doesn't have to be next to the ground.
- Rats and mice can slip through incredibly small openings. The skull bones of some species actually move to make it easier for them to get where they want to go. A house mouse can easily slip through a hole that is a half-inch in diameter.
- If you see mice droppings (small black oblong pellets that look like pieces of dirt), call a pest control expert who can evaluate your home and give you a plan for killing the existing mice and preventing them from coming back. Don't attempt to destroy the mice or remove traps yourself.
- The exterminator will likely use some type of rodenticide as part of the plan. If you have pets and children, make certain that the poison is placed where the kids and animals can't get it.
- Cabinets should be checked regularly for droppings. Don't vacuum up mice droppings; the dust is blown out of the back end of the vacuum into the air you're breathing. Instead, wet down all droppings with bleach or disinfectant. Use rubber gloves and discard all rags or material used to clean up the droppings.
- Don't replace insulation after a mouse infestation. Moving around the insulation sends dust and feces particles throughout your entire home through the ducts and ventilation system—and the systems often recycle the same

contaminated air. Leave the insulation alone. Some heating and air-conditioning companies will not send out cleanup crews until six months to a year has passed since the mice have been removed.

## HOT BUTTON

- Keep your house or apartment as crumb-free as possible to discourage uninvited guests.
- Remove all boxes and papers where roaches and mice like to live.
- Seal all small spaces.
- If you seem to have an infestation of any kind, contact an exterminator.

# Cougars (Mountain Lions)

Also known as puma, panther, and mountain lion, the cougar is typically a shy creature that avoids people and dines on elk, deer, and smaller mammals. Yet as people have encroached more and more into "mountain lion country," there have been an increasing number of attacks in recent years.

Once hunted nearly to extinction, cougars are on the rebound. The ban on sport hunting in California has helped to double their numbers in that state with present estimates of just over 5000 animals.

Starting in the late 1980s lion sightings became increasingly common, with some animals popping up in untraditional places. On the outskirts of Denver, mountain lions can be found in neighborhoods of $500,000 homes. In Montana, cougars have been seen hiding under boat docks or passing through rural yards at midday.

Cougars have killed eight people in North America (primarily in the West, where there's the highest cougar population) since

January 1971, more than they killed during the preceding 80 years. Most, but not all, victims have been children.

Cougars appear to be bolder now as they adjust to people hiking, camping, climbing, and skiing in their areas. Because cougar attacks are almost always directly linked to the need to satisfy hunger, there is some belief among experts that the juvenile cougars, who are looking for new territory are more likely to drift into populated areas and give human "bait" a try.

While the number of cougar attacks is less than many other dangers that could befall us, the nature of the attacks is horrifying. A 10-year-old child who runs ahead of his family on a well-traveled hiking trail in Rocky Mountain National Park is killed by a cougar; an 18-year-old jogger in Idaho Springs, Colorado, is mauled to death only a few hundred yards from his high school; a 40-year-old mother of two is killed while jogging on a road east of Sacramento. Because the situations are so "close to home" and so grisly, people are particularly aware of the need to be on guard.

## ABOUT COUGARS

Cougars are tawny-colored with black-tipped ears and tail, smaller than the jaguar, but one of North America's largest cats. They inhabit forested areas in the Western United States and a small section of Florida. Adult males may be more than eight feet long from nose to end of tail; they generally weigh between 130–150 pounds, and sometimes as much as 200 pounds. Females can be seven feet long and weigh between 65–90 pounds. They growl, purr, hiss, and scream, but cougars don't roar. Solitary animals, they usually hunt alone at night and prefer to ambush their prey from behind. They usually kill with a powerful bite below the base of the skull.

Cougars can sprint 40 miles per hour and leap 20 feet into a tree. The animals have good eyesight and a keen nose, so they know you're coming long before you're upon them.

## COUGAR-PROOF YOUR HOME

If you live in mountain lion country, some simple measures can reduce the likelihood of your property being a mountain lion's hunting grounds:

- To make it difficult for a mountain lion to approach your yard unseen, clear brush away from the house and yard. Install outdoor lighting, particularly along walkways.
- Don't put out salt blocks or hay to attract deer and elk, and don't feed your pets outdoors.
- Deer-proof your landscape. Avoid using plants that deer like. Check with your state department of fish and game for additional localized information on what you can do to co-exist peacefully with the cougars in your area.
- Keep pets secure by keeping them inside at night. If the animals are outside, they are safest in a kennel with a secure top.
- Keep livestock secure at night, preferably in enclosed sheds or barns.
- Don't let children play in the yard unwatched or alone.

## AVOIDING COUGAR CONFRONTATIONS

While bears are more likely to leave the "subservient" person alone, cougars respond in an opposite manner: the louder and more boorish you are, the more likely you are to be spared.

- Don't hike alone.
- Don't let children run ahead on the hiking trail.
- Make noise while hiking to make the cougar aware that you're coming.
- If you encounter a cougar, don't approach it. Give the animal time to escape.

- Don't try to outrun a cougar. This may stimulate its instinct to chase.
- If approached by a cougar, make eye contact, make a lot of noise, and try to look as large and forbidding as possible by raising your arms or opening your jacket while backing away. Be firm and loud about the fact that you are dangerous.
- Don't turn your back or curl up in a ball on the ground and play dead. You're a perfect victim then.
- If the animal ultimately attacks, fight back. Kick, punch, and yell. Try to remain standing and throw rocks, or whack the cougar with a stick, to persuade it you're not prey.
- Cougars usually attack the head and neck, so try to remain standing and facing the attacking animal. Don't do anything that involves crouching down (tying your shoe, picking up a child). To a cougar, you then look like a four-footed animal, and there's no reason not to go after you. If you need to pick up a child, bend your knees, keeping your back straight and keep your eyes on the cougar at all times.

## ONE TOP TIP TO TEACH CHILDREN ABOUT COUGARS

Because of their smaller size, children are more likely to be victims of cougars:

- When hiking, children should stay with the group. Running ahead can spell disaster.

## HOT BUTTON

- If confronted by a cougar, don't turn your back on him, and be as loud as possible. Lift your jacket up "like wings" to try to appear as large and threatening as possible.

- If you have a child with you, bend only at the knees, keeping your back straight, in order to pick up the child. Avoid crouching. Keep your eyes on the cougar at all times.

## Coyotes

What Native Americans called "little wolf" is nothing like the unfortunate Wile E. Coyote depicted in the Warner Bros. cartoons. *Canis latrans* would never find himself on the receiving end of a box of exploding dynamite. Today's "barking dog" is smart, extremely adaptable, and a true survivor. The call of the coyote—the melodious yips, barks, and howls that used to be heard primarily in desert areas—can now be heard in suburban backyards and city parks.

Though in parts of the West people may have encroached on coyote territory, that's only half of this man and beast story. The coyote is unusual because as a species it has decided to snuggle in and adapt to man; there have been recent sightings in disparate places ranging from Dayton to Denver, from Dallas to New York City's Central Park.

Wildlife experts have found that because the coyote is wily, intelligent, and highly adaptable, the very thought of trying to eradicate the species from an area is virtually impossible. Instead, communities are dealing with coyotes on a nuisance basis—if one particular animal is causing trouble, animal control specialists will try to locate and remove that animal.

Though pets sometimes fall victim to coyotes, coyotes are not usually considered dangerous to humans. However, recent attacks suggest that as coyote populations grow and spread throughout a community, attacks may become more frequent. Children are at more risk than adults, because they are smaller in size. In 1998 a little boy playing in his yard in Sandwich, Massachusetts, was attacked by a coyote; he was only freed after his mother pried the animal off her son. There have also been a series of incidents in Yellowstone that were nothing less than bizarre. In one case, a cross-country skier was knocked down and mauled by a coyote that apparently had lain in wait alongside the trail. In another incident, a road surveyor working in the park was attacked by a coyote that lunged for her throat and charged repeatedly before a fellow worker drove the animal off with rocks.

## ABOUT COYOTES

The coyote looks like a medium-sized dog and weighs from 20–50 pounds. Most are gray in color, but some show rust or brown coloration. They have a bushy tail that is tipped with black. The eastern coyote is larger, swifter, stronger, and more aggressive than its western and southwestern counterparts. This animal can weigh up to 50–60 pounds and somewhat resembles a German shepherd, although there are color variants. The coyote is omnivorous and eats fruits, grasses, and vegetables in addition to small mammals.

Coyotes contribute to the balance of nature by controlling the rodent population. Ranchers hate them because they kill sheep and poultry, though these domestic animals are not their primary diet.

Though the coyote is considered nocturnal, its habits depend largely on climate and habitat. Those that live in the desert tend to be more active at twilight and dawn when the temperature goes down. Those that live in temperate climates may forage during the daylight hours unless humans have harassed them. During winter when food is scarce, the coyote will hunt both day and night. In the summer they may nap during the day and find food at night.

## DEALING WITH URBAN COYOTES

It is becoming increasingly common for coyotes to attack family pets. Coyotes don't actively set out to hunt them, but if a coyote establishes a routine hunting pattern and finds that cats and small dogs are in the vicinity, the pets make an irresistible dinner offering. A repetition of this behavior over a period of time can cause some coyotes to fall into a pattern of seeking domestic animals.

- Don't feed pets outside as the food will attract coyotes and other nuisance wildlife.
- Don't leave pets outside unattended, especially at night. However, daylight is no longer a protection against coyotes, as some have been sighted during the day.

## TAKE PRECAUTIONS WITH CHILDREN IF COYOTES ARE IN THE AREA

- Don't leave young children outside unattended.
- Coyotes can carry rabies, so if there is any contact with the animal, the wound should be washed thoroughly with soap and water and the victim should be taken to the nearest medical facility for additional care.
  (Also see "Rabies.")
- If a coyote is posing a problem in your neighborhood, report it to the animal control department in your town or county.

## ONE TOP TIP TO TEACH CHILDREN ABOUT COYOTES

Encourage your children to tell you about any "stray" doglike animal they see.

## HOT BUTTON

- If coyotes are spotted in the area, step up your vigilance in protecting your pets and your children.
- Call an animal control officer if a coyote poses a threat to you or your neighbors.

# Dogs

Dogs have been a part of our society as working partners and household pets since the day of the cave dweller. Despite their long-term presence in our lives, few people have learned the equivalent of "nice to meet you" for dog encounters.

Dogs, like people, have unique personalities, fears, and moods. Catching a dog at a bad moment can often lead to a serious bite. The dog may be surprised or feel threatened and will try to protect itself—a natural response for an animal.

Dog bite victims are part of a largely unrecognized health concern. The number of dog bite injuries dwarfs the reported cases of mumps, measles, and whooping cough combined. While the increasing number of dogs bred for fighting is contributing to rising injury statistics, experts feel that the real explanation behind the numbers has to do with nothing more complicated than closer contact between people and dogs, and the inability of many people to properly train their pets.

Each year the Centers for Disease Control and Prevention estimates that 4.7 million people are bitten by dogs, 800,000 of them badly enough to require medical treatment. At least 60 percent of dog bites and 72 percent of fatal bites involve children. Children are the most common victims of severe dog bites, and since children are often bitten in the face (a convenient target for a dog), the treatment for many bites involves plastic surgery.

Knowing proper behavior, and teaching it to your children, can make encounters with friendly dogs all the more pleasurable, and it can save you from injury and your child from possible death when you meet up with a dog who is vicious.

## WISE BEHAVIOR AROUND DOGS

Most people (about 70 percent) are bitten by dogs they know. Though the neighbor's dog may seem as friendly as your own, all dogs must be treated with respect.

- Avoid dogs who do not have an owner nearby. Dogs in cars, behind fences, or tied up outside a store should be left alone; unfamiliar dogs running free with no owner in sight should be reported to the animal control center in your area. If it's a stray, it should be off the street; if it's lost, the owner will be delighted you found it.
- Before approaching any dog with an owner, both adults and children should ask permission to pet it.
- If the owner indicates the dog may be petted, extend a loose fist for the dog to sniff. Then pet the dog on its back rather than on the more sensitive ears or head.
- If a young child wants to pet a dog and permission has been granted, kneel down behind the child and extend your own fist along with his or hers. If the dog is wiggling with excitement, your body will provide some stability for the child, who could easily be overwhelmed by a large dog or a frisky animal.
- If you're visiting someone's home and the dog does not approach you, it's giving you a message—don't approach it. The dog may not be feeling well or may be very old, both of which may cause it to react unexpectedly.
- If you regularly walk or jog in an area where dogs run loose:

  ◆ Go with a buddy or buddies. Most dogs are reluctant to approach a group of people.

  ◆ Carry pepper spray, or one trainer recommends an umbrella. If approached, you may be able to pop open the umbrella and scare the dog away.

- Try to avoid startling any dog, even your own. If your approach is unexpected, the animal may respond aggressively, catching both of you by surprise.
- Don't tease any dog or bother it when it's eating, sleeping, chewing on something, or caring for puppies. These are "private" moments and should be respected.
- Always supervise when dogs and children are playing.

## WARNING SIGNS OF A DOG TO AVOID

Unless the dog is asleep, an animal usually gives clear signals to keep people away:

- A frightened dog can be dangerous. It may have its tail between its legs, with ears back. The fur may be standing on end.
- An angry dog usually barks or growls, showing its teeth. The tail may go back and forth slowly. People sometimes interpret this behavior as underlying friendliness, but the proverbial wagging tail isn't always what it seems. Look for other signs as well.

## IF YOU ARE APPROACHED BY AN AGGRESSIVE DOG

- Don't run away. The dog's natural instinct is to chase you.
- Don't yell or scream. If you're carrying something with you, toss it to the dog to divert it. Then *freeze*. Stand perfectly still with hands held close to the body. Don't yell or say anything and don't look at the animal. Dogs interpret direct eye contact as a threat or challenge. (Practice "acting like a

tree" with your children.) In all likelihood, the dog will find you dull and will go looking for something more interesting. If it doesn't, then start backing up slowly, talking calmly, and watching the animal at all times. If the dog persists, some experts say that if you can wrap your hand in a jacket, or something else you're wearing, you can try pushing into the dog's mouth as it comes at you. This forward punch by you will throw the dog off balance and may send it away.

## IF A DOG KNOCKS YOU DOWN OR IF A CHILD IS SITTING WHEN THREATENED

- Act like a rock. Roll into a fetal position with knees to the chest, elbows tucked in, and hands clasped behind the neck, protecting both your neck and your ears.

## IF YOU WITNESS A DOGFIGHT OR YOUR DOG IS ATTACKED

- Don't put yourself or any part of your body between the two dogs.
- If your dog is on a leash when attacked, drop the leash. Holding the leash will hamper your dog's ability to defend himself, and you may get pulled into the fray. If you get hurt, you're no use to your dog.
- If you have anything with you, try to put that item (a bike, a jacket, a rake, etc.) between the two dogs.
- If you have pepper spray or citronella spray, use it.
- If you are at home and your dog is attacked, use a water hose or a fire extinguisher to break up the fight. The chemicals in the fire extinguisher are irritating to the dogs but do no long-term damage.
- After an attack, take your dog to the vet. Even if he appears to be fine, he ought to be examined.

## IF SOMEONE IS BITTEN

- Immediately wash the wound thoroughly with soap and warm water.
- If the dog who attacked was unfamiliar to you, it will need to be located and checked for rabies. Call the local animal control agency or the police for help. If the owner can be located and a rabies vaccination certificate is produced, the victim won't have to get rabies shots.
- Contact a doctor for additional care and advice. If the victim's tetanus shot isn't current, a physician may want it updated.

## THREE TOP TIPS TO TEACH CHILDREN ABOUT DOGS

Children need to be taught to treat any animal with kindness and respect. Flailing at or pounding on a dog, pulling its ears, trying to climb on it or carry it, or in any way causing the dog distress is asking for trouble. Once children understand proper behavior around animals, the three most important safety messages to convey are these:

1. Always ask permission to approach and pet a dog.
2. Allow a dog to see and sniff you before petting it, then pet it on the back.
3. Act like a tree or a rock (if you're on the ground) if you're approached by a threatening dog.

## BEING A RESPONSIBLE OWNER

The job of raising a trustworthy dog is your responsibility. Once you become a pet owner, you must use good judgment and remain alert for situations that put your dog or other people at risk.

- Research the breed or the dog you select to bring into your home. A dog with aggressive tendencies doesn't belong in a home with children.
- Attend a training class with your puppy. The class will give you lessons on helping your dog act like a "good" dog.
- Socialize your dog by taking him with you as often as possible when he's young and familiarize him with different situations that involve all types of dogs and people, including children.
- If you have no plans to breed your dog, spay or neuter it. This procedure will reduce your dog's desire to roam and fight with other dogs. According to the Humane Society, neutering can reduce by three times the risk that your animal will bite someone.
- License your dog as required by law and provide regular veterinary care, including rabies vaccinations. Rabies vaccinations are recommended at 8–12 weeks, a booster at one year, and then regular shots at three-year intervals. If dogs are vaccinated, they are not able to spread the disease.
- A new type of medical identification device is now available for dogs. The ID system (Pet ID or Pet Scope) is a tiny plastic cylinder that contains a microdot and a magnifying lens that permits a viewer to read 25 lines of information about your dog—basic identification along with a list of current vaccinations, medical conditions, and any special information required. These IDs can be purchased at a pet store. You then fill out an information sheet, and mail it back to the manufacturer. There, the data is put on microfilm and sent back to you. You then insert the microfilm into the three-fourths inch cylinder, which can be attached to your animal's collar. With this ID, your dog is more likely to be returned to you, and if by any chance your dog bites anyone, the list of vaccinations will bring peace of mind to the victim.

- Don't play aggressive or "attack" games ("sic 'em") with your dog. Tug of war actually strengthens the jaw muscles, which is ill-advised.
- Teach your dog submissive behaviors such as rolling over to expose the abdomen. From puppyhood, work on making your dog relinquish food from its mouth without growling. This is a submissive behavior that will also permit you to remove dangerous "treats" like bones or parts of dead animals that your dog may pick up on walks or dig out of wastebaskets or garbage.
- Reward your dog for good behavior; punitive action is less effective and bites often follow harsh punishment.
- Be particularly alert when your dog is in a new situation or around people you don't know. The visitor to your home who flails his arms or decides to pick up your dog, or the toddler who follows your pet ceaselessly, are both acting in a manner to which your dog may not be accustomed. A dog's signal that its tolerance is being tested may be to snarl or bite.
- Some owners pet their dogs to calm them when the dog shows signs of aggression, such as barking or lunging at someone who comes to the front door. Instead of calming the pet, this actually reinforces the negative behavior. Instead, you must let him know you are displeased by removing the animal from the situation immediately.
- If your dog shows repeated signs of aggression, check with a vet, animal behaviorist, qualified dog trainer, or community animal care agency who may have suggestions.
- Err on the safe side. Always avoid stressful settings for your dog—anything from long car trips or big crowds to Fourth of July picnics that include fireworks.

# IF DESPITE YOUR BEST EFFORTS
# YOUR DOG BITES SOMEONE

- Confine the dog immediately and check on the victim.
- Help the victim as needed. Any dog bite should be seen by a physician, but you'll want to wash the wound and bandage it in the meantime.
- Provide the victim with a copy of your dog's rabies vaccination certificate.
- Cooperate with the animal control officer. If the dog must be quarantined for any length of time, ask if he can be confined with you at home or at your vet's hospital.
- In the eyes of the law, dogs are property, and you can be held liable for harm done by your dog. Exactly how the law affects you depends on the state in which you reside. Most homeowners' or renters' insurance policies cover the costs of dog-created damage or injury, but review your policy to be sure you have sufficient coverage. And keep in mind that if your dog does bite someone, you are at risk of the incident affecting your insurance coverage negatively. There has been a recent trend among companies to cancel the insurance, exclude future dog-related incidents from coverage, or significantly raise rates.
- Seek help to prevent the dog from biting again.
- If you can't control your dog's behavior, carefully consider what next step to take. If your dog is uncomfortable around children or dislikes other dogs, you may be able to place it in an environment where these stimuli are absent, and the new owner may be able to manage the situation. However, if your dog bites unpredictably, you may have few options but to have it destroyed before it hurts someone else very seriously.

## HOT BUTTON

- Even a sweet dog you know can be startled, so always give dogs an opportunity to realize you're there.
- Don't subject your own dog to a persistent toddler, big crowds, or anything to which he isn't accustomed. Don't take the chance that the stress will become too much for him.

# Killer Bees and Other Stinging Insects

When sightings of the first "killer bee" in the United States, near Brownsville, Texas, were first announced in 1990, many residents feared they would be attacked by a swarm of "killers" the moment they walked out the door.

Nothing could be farther from the truth. While an attack by a swarm of killer bees would be quite serious, killer bees only attack to defend. If you leave them alone, they'll leave you alone. Killer bees get their name from the fact that if angered, an entire swarm may attack a person, leaving hundreds of bites. As many as 2,000 stings have been reported on one person.

Statistically, stings from Hymenoptera (bees, wasps, yellow jackets, hornets, and stinging ants) can be just as dangerous as an attack by killer bees. That's because a relatively high number of people have immediate and catastrophic allergic reactions to the insect venom. About 50 Americans die each year as a result of stings, and up to a million Americans are so allergic that a single sting can be deadly.

But first things first. The story behind the arrival of the killer bee is a good one.

# THE KILLER BEE

What we call the "killer bee" was brought to this hemisphere in the 1950s.

Before European settlers arrived on this continent, there weren't any honeybees at all in the U.S. In the 1600s, Europeans introduced the honeybee to this continent, and as a result, the "everyday" variety of honeybee in America is also referred to as a "Europeanized bee." As the honey industry spread south into Latin America, beekeepers discovered that the Europeanized bees didn't do very well in hot sticky climates. For that reason, about fifty years ago some Brazilians imported a batch of honeybees from Africa, nicknamed "killer bees" because they are more aggressive than their European cousins. The Brazilians assumed that by crossbreeding the two they could create European honeybees that could survive in the tropics.

But like a bad horror movie, a bunch of African bees escaped and started breeding and spreading northward, propagating their aggressive behavior. They became media worthy in the United States as they moved northward into Texas and New Mexico.

Though the Africanized honeybees have spread 200–300 miles a year in the parts of the country where the temperatures are warm, they're not "snow bunnies." On occasion and totally by accident, Africanized bees have been transported from Texas or Mexico to Maine, but after a month or two of cold weather they die. While they may eventually adapt to colder climates, there's no doubt that their movement north has been slowed by their discomfort in cold weather.

African bee venom is the same as that of the domestic bee, and a single sting from an African bee is no more dangerous than that of a honeybee. However, killer bees can be quite vicious when upset. Like other bees, they're busy with the tasks ahead of them, but if their hive is disturbed, or someone attacks them with swatters or bug bombs, they react as a unit, making a massive attack.

Unlike the domestic honeybee that prefers living in clean, dry, high areas like hollow trees and walls, Africanized honeybees dwell in small areas—underground cavities, flower pots, old tires, and birdhouses. If you think killer bees have arrived in your area, contact a pest control officer.

## WHAT TO DO IF YOU ARE ATTACKED BY "KILLER BEES"

- "Run like the devil," say the experts. Most people, particularly when fueled by adrenaline, can run faster than bees can fly, and since bees just want to defend their territory, they'll eventually give up the chase because they accomplished what they needed to.
- Aside from running, button up any clothing you're wearing and close your mouth. A bee can sting the back of the throat, causing the airway to swell shut.
- If you're near water, jump in to confuse them. The water will wash off the odor left on you by the first sting—the element that is attracting and provoking the rest of the swarm to attack.

## THE HONEYBEE

Honeybees are light golden brown, and their bodies are covered in fuzz. The stinger of the honeybee consists of a needlelike shaft to which is attached a bulb-like poison sac. The shaft has a sheath covering two darts whose job it is to open a wound so that the poison can be injected. If you catch the wound in time, you can limit the amount of poison that goes into the wound. Because their stingers are "single-use" equipment, a victim can at least have the satisfaction of knowing the bee died after the sting was made.

## YELLOW JACKETS AND WASPS

An encounter with a yellow jacket, wasp, or hornet can be nasty because these insects can sting again and again. If one is buzzing around you, resist the urge to kill it—squashing its venom sac releases a chemical that incites others to seek revenge.

Experts say that yellow jackets have the capacity to learn, which can prove particularly unpleasant for people. These insects learn where to find good food (picnic tables, for example), and they also learn what time the food will be there. Don't expect to see them at 8:00 A.M.; they'd prefer to wait until noon.

Several types of bees and wasps dwell in the ground and attack lawn mowers (and the people operating them) when the mowing disturbs their nests. The most common ground-dweller is the yellow jacket wasp. They live in large underground colonies. If your yard has yellow jackets, you might try mowing in the evening or early morning when the wasps aren't active, and be sure to wear protective clothing. Or you may want to eliminate the wasp home. Watch for the hole the wasps are using. Apply insecticide to the hole. Check with a gardening store about what is best to use in your area, and follow the directions carefully.

## FIRE ANTS

Killer bees aren't the only dangerous insect to arrive from South America. Their cousin, the fire ant, is more widespread in the United States, more destructive, and so far deadlier. These antagonistic ants have ruined picnics, forced the cancellation of high school football games, and kept children out of their yards because of their painful stings.

Unfortunately, fire ants aren't even helpful to the environment. They throw off the ecosystem because they crowd out or kill many other insects, causing lizards, birds, and small mammals to move away. The ants are strangely attracted to electric currents, and have been known to chew through underground cables, disrupting everything from telephone service to airport runway lights, and even starting fires.

Fire ants first appeared in Mobile, Alabama, in the 1930s, probably coming in from South America on shiploads of lumber. They are now well established throughout the South with a few isolated pockets farther north in places such as Virginia, and on the West Coast as far north as Washington. While cold weather has previously killed them off, they are beginning to adapt to colder temperatures, and they may well make inroads into the Midwest and Northeast.

In many cases, ants grasp the skin with their mandibles in order to anchor themselves for the insertion of their stingers. Some stinging ants cannot sting at all unless they can grasp the skin.

## HOW TO AVOID BEING STUNG OR BITTEN

- Don't wear bright flowery clothing, or scents associated with soaps, perfumes, and lotions. These serve to attract stinging insects.
- When spending time near flowers and fruits, wear long pants and long-sleeved shirts and shoes (not sandals).
- Cover food and drinks at picnics, and don't drink from cans. Wasps are attracted to sweet drinks and may climb into a can for a taste, giving anyone who drinks from the can an unfortunate surprise.
- Don't swat at stinging insects.
- Watch for hives on your property. If you find one, hire a professional to take it down.

## WHAT TO DO IF STUNG

- The stinger of the bee will remain embedded in your skin, and the faster you get it out, the less severe the sting will be. Use a needle, the edge of a credit card, or your fingernail to try to scrape out the stinger. By getting it out quickly, you may be able to remove it before all the venom is released into your skin.
- Wash the sting site with soap and water.
- Relieve pain by rubbing an aspirin tablet into the moist skin where you received the bite. Some people mix meat tenderizer or baking soda into water and use that solution to soothe the sting. Ice also helps temporarily.
- After bites from yellow jackets and wasps, watch for signs of secondary infections. They are scavengers, and you may see some additional infection as a result.
- If you're bitten while exercising, slow down immediately so you can pay attention to the sting.
- Even if you seem fine immediately afterward, tell someone you've been stung. That way, if you have any type of reaction in a few minutes, that person will know what happened to you.

## RECOGNIZING AN ALLERGIC REACTION

A normal response to insect bites or stings involves a localized reaction in the form of pain and itching, and a weal (the swelling of the bite).

If the swelling intensifies, feels hot, and does not go away, a physician should be consulted. There may be a secondary infection. If the swelling includes joints or an entire limb, the possibility of an allergy should be investigated.

An allergic reaction (anaphylactic reaction) to an insect sting often begins with a dry, hacking cough and a sense of constriction in the throat and chest. The eyes may begin to itch and the area around the eyes swell. Hives, sneezing, wheezing, and either paleness or flushing may accompany these initial symptoms. The victim's pulse may become rapid, and the blood pressure may fall. If the reaction is severe, symptoms may progress rapidly to any combination of the following: nausea and vomiting, dizziness, faintness, cyanosis (bluish color of the lips, ears, and fingertips), laryngeal stridor (funny breathing sounds due to closing off the breathing tube, the trachea), chills and fever, collapse, incontinence, unconsciousness, and bloody, frothy sputum.

## GETTING IMMEDIATE TREATMENT

A particular danger presented by an insect allergy is how little time there may be to respond. A fatal systemic reaction can take place within two minutes.

A simple injection of epinephrine, if received in time, can arrest this reaction. If symptoms are not relieved, a second injection may be needed within 15–20 minutes along with injectable antihistamines.

Anyone who suffers a mild systemic reaction following a bee sting or the bite of any other insect should check with a physician for protective measures against a more serious reaction in the future.

## IF YOU'RE ALLERGIC

Anyone who has suffered symptoms of a systemic reaction or a severe local reaction should carry an antihistamine and an adrenaline kit and get an ID bracelet that lists your personal allergens. If you're stung, look for medical help immediately.

If given an EpiPen, a syringe filled with epinephrine (adrenaline) that can be injected into the thigh, read the directions and learn how to use it long before you need it. Carry it with you whenever you're going to be outdoors.

There are differences among the venoms secreted by various insects. A person who is sensitive to the stings of one may be only mildly bothered by another. However, in general, try to avoid being stung by anything at all.

What if you're stung by something but you're not sure it's the one to which you're allergic? If you sense the beginning of a reaction, treat yourself anyway. The side effects of the EpiPen are palpitations, tremor, anxiety, and possibly a slight elevation in blood pressure. Although these are rather uncomfortable symptoms, they aren't dangerous, and they are obviously less of a problem than an untreated anaphylactic episode. (People with major heart disease or arrhythmia should remind their allergist of this health history. The doctor should prescribe an EpiPen with a lower dosage and will review with the patient exactly what symptoms merit use of the EpiPen.)

If you've suffered a severe reaction, most allergists recommend that you undergo tests to identify the exact cause and then go through immunotherapy—a series of injections that will build up a basic immunity. According to the American Academy of Allergy, Asthma and Immunology (AAAAI), venom immunotherapy prevents future allergic reactions in 97 percent of treated patients.

## THREE TOP TIPS TO TEACH CHILDREN ABOUT STINGING INSECTS

1. Children should be taught not to disturb hives and to stay away from garbage cans where bees or wasps are flying.
2. If any family member—adult or child—is allergic, all family members should understand the importance of getting immediate help.
3. Talk to your child about how to scrape out a stinger. If they

can learn to do it themselves, they can save themselves a great deal of pain.

## HOT BUTTON

- If you are attacked by killer bees, run as fast as you can while covering as much of yourself with clothing as possible and being sure to close your mouth.
- If anyone in the family is allergic, be sure they carry an EpiPen.
- If you're stung, tell someone so they can help if you suffer a reaction.
- If you're with someone who has been stung and seems to be having an allergic reaction, seek medical help with all speed.

# Sharks

While *Jaws* certainly became a much bigger sensation than any movie called *Stinger* would have been, you have a greater chance of dying from a bee sting than you do of being eaten by a shark. Nonetheless, the 9-year-old child who was killed off the coast of Florida in 1998 by a tiger shark, and the experienced 42-year-old California sea-urchin diver who was attacked when he was treading water next to his boat while taking off some of his gear, makes one realize that "less likely" doesn't mean "impossible."

During the early part of this decade, the number of unprovoked shark attacks grew at a steady rate, rising from 36 in 1990 to an all-time high of 72 in 1995. More recently, the number has declined, with 40 unprovoked attacks recorded in 1996, 57 in 1997, and 49 in 1998.

Most likely because of the surface kicking and splashing that accompanies surfing, surfers were the most targeted recreational group worldwide, accounting for 69 percent of all 1998 shark attacks.

To a large extent, sharks are scavengers that eat injured fish, carrion, garbage, and other waste from ships as well as animals such as seals, turtles, birds, whales, crabs, and a wide range of fish. Scientists say that in the ocean, sharks perform the same vital function as predators and scavengers that carnivores do on land. By preying on weak or poorly adapted fish and marine mammals, sharks ensure that only the animals that are strong and healthy survive to reproduce.

Unfortunately, sharks themselves are under attack, which worries ecologists. Excessive hunting for their fins, meat, skins, and other valuable products could lead to the extinction of some species. Great whites have already been declared endangered in South Africa and parts of Australia, and the populations of several other species have been reduced to a point where recovery is very much in question.

## ABOUT SHARKS

There are 380 known species of sharks ranging from lantern sharks, which are about 8 inches long, to whale sharks, which can grow to 49 feet. Sharks have an acute sense of smell, but their vision, badly needed for hunting, is less acute.

Only 10 or 12 species have been known to ever hassle a human. Of those that are considered dangerous—the great white, the tiger shark, the bull shark, the hammerhead, and the blue shark—most live in very cold, deep waters, so not many divers ever see them.

When hunting for a good dinner, a shark can spend half an hour or more inspecting its prey, circling repeatedly, and making several dummy runs before choosing to bite. This large fish then kills using the "bite and spit" method. Because they prey on seals and sea lions, who can do a lot of damage with their huge claws, sharks generally bite once and then wait for their prey to die. The last thing a shark wants to do is risk injury to itself by attempting to eat an animal while it's still alive. A white shark whose vision is compromised is a dead white shark. Most humans survive attacks because they are with a buddy who pulls them from the water before the shark returns for his meal.

## "IT WAS AN ACCIDENT!"

Current theory holds that with rare exceptions, sharks don't intentionally attack human beings. Some attacks are probably cases of mistaken identity. Photographs have demonstrated that when seen underwater a person on a surfboard silhouetted against the sun is indistinguishable from a sea lion; a clumsy human swimming in murky water could easily be taken for a wounded fish; a scuba diver wearing a black wet suit and black fins may well appear to a passing shark to be an acceptable meal—a sea lion, perhaps. Unfortunately, by the time a shark takes a bite out of you, it's a little late for him to apologize for making the mistake.

If you've ever been on a beach that was cleared because sharks were in the area, then you'll be wise to learn how not to become bait.

## DON'T ACT LIKE BAIT

- Swim at beaches that are under the surveillance of lifeguards, who will close the beach if they see a shark, barracuda, or any other predator. Swim close enough to the lifeguard stations that you're aware as soon as a warning is sounded.
- Swim with a group, and don't go out too far. Sharks are less likely to come in toward beaches, particularly if the shark senses a lot of movement.

- If diving, get in and out of the boat quickly to avoid hanging out mid-water or on the surface "looking like an elephant seal."
- If you get cut or are retrieving anything that is bleeding, get out of the water as quickly as possible. Sharks are attracted to blood.
- If you see a shark while swimming, do not panic. Try to splash as little as possible, swimming with slow, steady strokes. Then leave the water as calmly as possible.
- If you're scuba diving, move to the bottom against a rock so you're protected from behind. You might also try to scare the shark away by releasing a stream of bubbles from your regulator.
- If the shark attacks, punch it or poke it sharply in the snout, eye, or gills. Like other animals, sharks are sensitive around the nose, and a good punch in that area may send it away. Because the shark will only bite once, the more you can do to lessen the impact of that first bite, the better chance your swimming or diving buddies will have of getting you out of the water and to medical care in time to save you. If you're bitten, the odds are in your favor that you'll survive.

## ONE TOP TIP TO TEACH CHILDREN ABOUT SHARKS

Always swim at beaches with lifeguards and heed any warnings they give.

## HOT BUTTON

- If you spot a shark while you're in the water, swim away from the animal, splashing as little as possible.
- If the shark comes close enough to attack, fight back and try to bop it on the nose, in the gills, or poke it in the eyes.

# Snakes

If you were bitten by a snake a hundred and fifty years ago, the recommended "cure" might have killed you if the snakebite didn't. During the nineteenth century it was believed that extremely large doses of alcohol would neutralize the venom in the snakebite. By 1908 suspicions about this "treatment" finally led to an investigation, and at that time it was estimated that as many as 5 percent of all "snakebite" deaths were actually from overdoses of alcohol. In one instance a fellow had been bitten by a harmless nonvenomous snake and died later of acute alcohol poisoning.

Treatments didn't get much better when the medical community gave up the alcohol "cure." In 1895 doctors were testing the effectiveness of repeated injections of strychnine an excellent rat poison that inevitably kills people, too. By World War I, snakebite kits contained potassium permanganate crystals, which were to be rubbed into the wound—a treatment akin to rubbing dirt into the bite.

Treating snakebites has remained a medical backwater, plagued by outmoded theories, ambitious quacks, and major misjudgments. Today, using a tourniquet and cutting the bite to suck out the venom has also fallen out of favor, yet medical advances reveal no sure cure.

The most powerful snakebite weapon used today is antivenin serum, which is made by repeatedly injecting venom into horses (or sometimes sheep) until they develop a resistance. Then the blood is drawn and processed into a serum, complete with impurities from the horse. Because of a high incidence of allergic reaction to the antivenin, it must be used only under careful medical supervision.

In the United States, about 8,000 people per year receive venomous bites, and 9–15 victims die. Most bites are from pit vipers—rattlesnakes, copperheads, and cottonmouths—that live in southern states.

Other countries see quite different statistics, with about 15,000 people per year in India dying from bites from the krait, a snake whose venom is deadly enough to kill an elephant. A best guess places the number of snakebite deaths worldwide each year at more than 50,000.

Every state but Maine, Hawaii, and Alaska is home to at least one of twenty domestic poisonous snake species. People who hike, picnic, or camp in the wilderness as well as those who live in snake-inhabited areas should be aware of the potential dangers posed by poisonous snakes.

## ABOUT SNAKES

Two families of venomous snakes are native to the United States. About 99 percent of the venomous bites in this country are from pit vipers (of the family *Crotalidae*), which include rattlesnakes, copperheads, and cottonmouths (water moccasins). These snakes are referred to as pit vipers because of a small heat-sensitive pit between the eye and nostril that allows the snake to sense its prey at night. The jaws of these snakes can open alarmingly wide, making the bite from this species more likely to hit its target.

The other family of domestic poisonous snakes is *Elapidae*, which includes two species of coral snakes found chiefly in the southern states. These are related to the very dangerous Asian cobras and kraits. All coral snakes in the U.S. can be identified by a particular color sequence: "Red in black, venom lack; red on yellow, kill a fellow." While their poison is lethal, often causing respiratory paralysis, their smaller mouth makes it harder for them to be as effective when biting a human.

Because snakes have no capacity to chew their food, the venom serves as a strong saliva to break down and allow the snake to digest whatever it has bitten or eaten. Venom is often classified in two major categories: neurotoxic (nerve-affecting) and hemotoxic (blood-affecting). The neurotoxin produces respiratory failure or suppresses the heart action, and it circulates more quickly; the hemotoxin destroys blood cells and other tissues and spreads more slowly.


## AVOID SNAKES WHEN POSSIBLE

Most snakebites are highly preventable. The snake doesn't want to have anything to do with you, so unless you put yourself in a position to tangle with it, people and snakes can coexist peacefully:

- If you're in the wilderness, know how you would travel to the nearest hospital. This is actually important preparation in case of any kind of on-the-trail emergency.
- Most bites occur on the feet and legs, so wear thick leather boots and full-length denim jeans for hiking, and be conscious of where you step.
- Try to stay on hiking paths and trails, avoiding tall grass as much as possible.
- If you encounter a snake, leave it alone and don't try to catch it. Walk around the snake, giving it a berth of about six feet. Ninety percent of the wounds on women and children occur on a foot or ankle; among males over age 15, 90 percent of the bites occur on an upper extremity, usually a hand or arm. Since snakes don't generally jump that high, scientists conjecture that this can be attributed to the "Pecos Bill Syndrome." This is a condition that occurs when testosterone, machismo, and often alcohol come into play and lead the fellow to pick up the snake or even try to kiss it.
- Keep your hands and feet out of areas you can't see and be as careful as possible when rock climbing.
- Don't hike at night—it's the prime time for snakes to be out. If you must be out at night, carry a flashlight and wear boots.

- Snakes like warm places, so check your sleeping bag at night and your shoes in the morning for "surprises."
- If someone kills a snake, or you find one you think is dead, don't pick it up. Two toxicologists in Phoenix found that 15 percent of the rattlesnake bites they treated in a ten-month period came from snakes that had been decapitated, shot, or beaten until dead. Dr. Jeffrey R. Suchard of the Good Samaritan Regional Medical Center and his colleague Dr. Frank LoVecchio started the study in 1997, after they saw a patient who'd been bitten by the corpse of a snake. Five of the 34 rattlesnake-bite victims they treated were all bitten by dead snakes. Two of the snakes were even decapitated, but reflex action made the head bite the victim. In one case, the bite was so damaging that the person's finger eventually had to be amputated.

## WHAT TO DO IF BITTEN

Because it is difficult to positively identify a snake, anyone who is bitten should seek medical care promptly. Even a bite from a nonpoisonous snake can cause an infection or allergic reaction in some people. Victims can't afford to assume that the bite was from a nonvenomous snake.

- The Red Cross recommends the following:

  - Wash the bite with soap and water.
  - Immobilize the bitten area and keep it lower than the heart; keep the victim as calm as possible. You don't want to do anything that speeds the spread of the venom through the body.

- If you're more than a half hour away from medical treatment, then a bandage, wrapped two to four inches above the bite, may help slow the venom. The bandage should not be fastened as a tourniquet. Too many people have lost limbs from the reduced blood flow caused by a tourniquet. Make the band loose enough that a finger can slip under it.

- Today snakebite kits contain a suction instrument (the Sawyer Extractor), which can be placed over the bite to help draw venom out of the wound without making additional cuts. Use this if you are not able to get medical help right away. Don't make an incision in the bite area.

## SNAKEBITE SYMPTOMS

Symptoms vary by species. Rattlesnakes, copperheads, and water moccasins inject venom that destroys blood vessels; the victim will experience immediate sharp pain and swelling. If a lot of venom has been injected, discoloration of the tissue will also occur and the person may feel dizzy, nauseated and go into shock.

The bite of the coral snake may not cause immediate pain, but its venom attacks the central nervous system, paralyzing vital organs such as the lungs; so it's very important to get medical treatment right away.

The degree of seriousness of any snakebite depends on a combination of factors: the toxicity of the venom itself (some, like the Mojave rattlesnake, carry a neurotoxic venom that can affect the brain or spinal cord), how quickly medical care can be obtained, and the size of both the snake and the victim. In addition, sometimes (20–30 percent of pit viper bites and 60 percent of coral snakebites), no venom is injected, making a bite from a poisonous snake less harmful. It is still a bite, however, and will require treatment.

## TREATMENT

Building on the progress made by Louis Pasteur, who worked out the concept of immunity to the rabies virus, in 1887 Henry

Sewall developed a method of using a small amount of venom to protect a victim against the dangers of the venom of a bite.

Antivenins are the only effective treatment for some types of snakebite, and though they have a reasonably good safety record, there have been some life-threatening reactions to the antivenin. People who have an allergic reaction can go into ana-phylactic shock (the same reaction that kills 50–100 Americans a year from bee and wasp stings). However, because epinephrine (adrenaline), antihistamines, and resuscitation can be used effectively against anaphylactic shock, the current medical thinking is that a well-equipped intensive care unit can overcome allergic shock more easily than the complications resulting from a dose of poisonous venom.

At a hospital or medical center, professionals will generally administer a skin test to determine sensitivity. Some victims can be desensitized through a more gradual dispensing of the antivenin.

While new types of anitvenins are being developed, and some derived from sheep show promise for being safer to use, it is still important to be monitored by medical personnel throughout the process.

## THREE TOP TIPS TO TEACH CHILDREN ABOUT SNAKES

1. Don't try to catch snakes.
2. If you find a dead snake, don't pick it up. It can still bite you even when it's dead.
3. If you do get bitten, tell someone right away.

## HOT BUTTON

- Wear protective clothing, and give a wide berth to any snake.
- Don't hike at night. This is when you're most likely to encounter snakes.
- Get medical help right away for anyone who has been bitten. Snakebites aren't always painful, and sometimes people wait. Delay often cancels the opportunity for effective treatment.

# Spiders

Spiders are all around us, and bites from most types will result in nothing more serious than a localized reaction. You might need some type of lotion to soothe the itching or stinging, or if there are multiple bites, a bath in cornstarch or baking soda will help. A doctor may recommend taking an oral antihistamine to further arrest the reaction.

However, there are two types of spiders in the United States that are poisonous—the black widow and the brown recluse. The bites of both are potentially deadly if not treated quickly.

## ABOUT THE BLACK WIDOW

Only the female black widow is poisonous. She is just under half an inch long with an hourglass-shaped red-orange mark on her abdomen and a companion spot toward her rear end. If viewed from the topside, small dots of color (the sides of the hourglass) are detectable.

This spider is generally found in heavy vegetation, spinning her web under logs or in stone crevices, and is not usually aggressive.

The black widow packs more poison in every drop of venom than any other creature in North America. Fortunately, the black widow's bite sends out only a small amount of venom, and only two to four people a year die from it. The victims are almost always the very young, the very old, or the very allergic.

## WHAT TO DO IF BITTEN

If bitten, you may not feel the bite. There may be a little redness and swelling at first, and a small, red, slightly hard bump may form later. Other symptoms generally appear within 10–60 minutes if treatment is not begun. Headache, nausea, vomiting, dizziness, and heavy sweating may occur, and the victim may feel burning or numbness in his or her feet. The person may also suffer muscle spasms, stomach cramps, and chest pain that feels like a heart attack.

- Keep victim as calm as possible.
- Get to the nearest medical center quickly. Generally painkillers and observation are the first course of treatment, though a medical professional will be prepared to use an antivenin if necessary.

In virtually all cases, there will be a complete recovery.

## ABOUT THE BROWN RECLUSE

This brownish or sometimes reddish spider poses more of a risk to humans than the black widow, and both the male and female are dangerous. It has a black fiddle-shaped mark on its back, and does not spin a web but lurks in dark, quiet places such as closets or behind furniture as well as in forests. It is usually less than three-eighths of an inch long with unusually long legs. It attacks more readily in warmer months, usually at night and only when disturbed.

## WHAT TO DO IF BITTEN

As with most spiders, the bite of the recluse is often painless when it occurs, but within one to five hours there is a painful red blister. Intense pain will follow. A "bull's eye" lesion—a bluish circle around the blister with a red circle around that—usually develops. (The bite often leaves a lasting scar where the cells of the skin have been destroyed by venom.) The victim may suffer from chills, fever, generalized weakness, and a rash. Death has occurred in children when recluse venom caused fatal complications in the circulatory system.

- Use cold to reduce pain at the site if the victim is suffering.
- Get to the nearest medical center quickly, even if you only suspect a brown recluse bite. Treatment—consisting of cortisone, antihistamines, and antibiotic therapy—needs to be started immediately, particularly if the victim is a child.

## TWO TOP TIPS TO TEACH CHILDREN ABOUT SPIDERS

1. Some spiders are poisonous, and if bitten, your child should be taught to tell an adult.
2. Teach children to recognize the hourglass of the black widow and the fiddleback marking of the longish-legged brown recluse. Tell them to avoid these spiders, or to come and get you if they are worried.

## HOT BUTTON

- If someone is bitten by a spider and you know it was a black widow or brown recluse, seek medical help right away.
- Learn what a poisonous bite might look like: The brown recluse bite will develop a bluish circle around it; the bite of the black widow will be a small hard red bump. If

someone becomes ill and has suffered a bite, get the victim to a medical facility immediately to get an expert opinion on whether the bite and the illness are connected.

# Encephalitis and West Nile-like Virus

In the autumn of 1999 a medical mystery was "serialized" on the front page of New York metropolitan newspapers as the facts about a new mosquito-borne illness were gradually revealed. As large numbers of birds in the area died, and smaller numbers of people (mostly the elderly) were sickened and a few died, medical specialists worked to unravel the mystery about what was going on. Personnel from the Centers for Disease Control, the U.S. Army Medical Research Institute for Infectious Diseases and a pathologist at the Bronx Zoo were all involved.

When the Centers for Disease Control were first contacted about the human deaths in the New York City area, they originally tested the samples against diseases that were known to already exist in the United States. A close match was found with St. Louis encephalitis, a mosquito-borne illness that crops up in this country from time to time. However, as Dr. Tracey S. McNamara, head of pathology for the Wildlife Conservation Society (Bronx Zoo), thought about it, this conclusion began to puzzle her. Shortly before these deaths were reported, she had noticed an unusual number of birds dying in and around the zoo. Reports from neighboring communities of the death of crows in the area made her begin to think that the coincidence between the bird deaths and the human deaths was too great to ignore.

After running tests on bird samples at the National Veterinary Services Laboratory in Ames, Iowa, and prevailing upon a contact at the U.S. Army lab to run some additional tests for her, Dr. McNamara was able to approach the CDC again with the specifics. This new disease wasn't St. Louis encephalitis as originally thought but a virus never before seen in the Western Hemisphere, the West Nile-like virus.

At this writing, the experts are now focusing on two questions: Will the chemical spraying of communities to rid them of mosquitoes stem the spread of the disease? And how did the disease arrive in this country?

The public can rest assured that specialists will be working hard to find the answers.

## HOW IT IS TRANSMITTED

Both encephalitis and the West Nile-like virus are carried by birds and transmitted to people and other animals by mosquitoes. Those at greatest risk are the elderly, the young, and those with suppressed immune systems. The probability of infection is generally low because the mosquitoes that carry the diseases frequently don't transmit it. (With St. Louis encephalitis, only one bite in 300 from infected mosquitoes actually passes on the disease.) Because the transmission rate is low, there is no reason to panic over a single mosquito bite.

## SYMPTOMS

Many who get some form of encephalitis or the West Nile-like virus show few symptoms beyond a mild case of the flu. Severe infections can result in high fever, loss of consciousness, lethargy, brain damage, and death.

## TREATMENT

There is no cure but patients can be made more comfortable because symptoms can be treated. Patients recover when the immune system makes enough antibodies to destroy the virus.

## PRECAUTIONS

As always, prevention is the best cure:

- During an alert, avoid going out when the mosquitoes are at their most active: from about one hour before sundown until one hour after sunrise.
- Wear pants and long sleeves if you have to be out during a time when mosquito bites are common.
- Use insect repellents containing the chemical DEET.

## HOT BUTTON

- Take precautions when going out at times when mosquitoes are most active.
- Stay tuned for new facts about this newly identified disease.

# Hantavirus Pulmonary Syndrome

In 1993, when the Centers for Disease Control and Prevention was confronted with the deaths of several formerly healthy young people who happened to live in the Southwest on Indian reservations, they were baffled. Amazingly, the first people who died were long-distance runners in the best of health. Because the disease was particularly virulent (people died of adult respiratory distress within 24 hours) and puzzling, the CDC was determined to get a handle on it as soon as possible.

For one CDC sleuth, the key to working quickly involved working on-site and trying to involve the locals in identifying the source of the illness. As he talked to people in the area, the Native Americans on the reservation quickly sent him to medicine men, who were able to provide the clue the CDC needed to make a quick and accurate diagnosis: The medicine men had seen this type of disease in their people three times in the last

100 years. It always came during an exceptional pine nut harvest. The large quantity of pine nuts was accompanied by an exploding population of mice. Each time these elements were present, there was also human sickness.

Based on this lead, scientific testing quickly identified the disease as a hantavirus. This illness was originally discovered during the Korean War when thousands of United Nations soldiers developed fever, headache, hemorrhage, and sudden kidney failure after exposure to Korean field mice.

Hantavirus has now been identified in 25 states from New Mexico to Pennsylvania. It's one of the few viruses that can be transferred from rodents to humans through tiny droplets of urine, bits of freshly shed feces, or in the dust and dirt that gets stirred up and then inhaled. It can also be transmitted from human to human.

## SYMPTOMS

Early symptoms include fatigue, fever, and muscle aches. There may also be headaches, dizziness, chills, and nausea or abdominal pain. These can come from one to five days after exposure. Later, patients start coughing and experience shortness of breath.

If caught very early, hantavirus can be cured, but if it is not identified and addressed quickly, chances of recovery are poor.

## RISK ELEMENTS

Anything that puts you in contact with rodent droppings, urine, or nesting materials can cause exposure to the virus. Hiking, camping, cleaning out a summer cabin that has been closed up for the winter, or cleaning up around your own home can all put you at risk.

Construction workers and people in professions such as

plumbing or heating, ventilating, and air conditioning work are at risk from crawling around in areas where mice may have been.

## PREVENTION

The key to prevention is to eliminate or minimize contact with rodents. Recommendations from the Centers for Disease Control can be summed up as "Air out, seal up, trap up, and clean up" to prevent the disease. See "Cockroaches, Mice, and Rats" for specific suggestions.

If you live in an area where the deer mouse is likely to live, then you ought to take precautions whether or not you've seen droppings.

# Lyme Disease

Lyme disease is a bacterial infection that is carried through the bite of the deer tick, which thrives in areas where the weather is moist. The deer tick most commonly feeds from May through August and is generally found near wooded, brush-filled, grassy areas. However, you are also at risk in your own backyard.

This disease was first recognized in Lyme, Connecticut, in 1975 and is now the most common tick-borne illness in the United States. The disease is most prevalent in the Northeast and upper Midwest and in northern California and southern Oregon, but it has also been reported throughout the country as well as in Europe and parts of Asia and Australia.

Because the deer tick is so difficult to see—young ones are about the size of a poppy seed or the head of a pin, and the adults are no bigger than a grape seed—and because the bite is generally painless, people often don't know they've been bitten. In addition, symptoms can be mistaken for those of other diseases. Sometimes people don't get recognizable symptoms for months or even years.

Left untreated, the disease can lead to more severe problems such as chronic arthritis and cardiac or central nervous system abnormalities.

## SYMPTOMS

Typically Lyme disease causes a bull's eye rash, flu-like symptoms, and headaches. Muscle and joint pain may also occur. Scientists have learned that toothaches are sometimes a symptom of Lyme disease.

## DIAGNOSIS

Through 1999, diagnosis of Lyme disease was made via a blood test that registered antibody levels. The problem with this testing method is that it can't be used during the earliest stage of the disease because antibody levels are too low to be detected, and the test also can't distinguish between vaccine antibodies or antibodies created because of the presence of disease.

In late 1999, medical researchers writing in the *Journal of the American Medical Association* reported a breakthrough. There is now a new way to tell if a person has Lyme disease as early as a week after a tick bite, several weeks earlier than the current test. The new test is also a big improvement over the old one because it can distinguish between active and past infection and between active infection and vaccination.

## TREATMENT

If detected in time, Lyme disease can usually be treated with oral antibiotics. The majority of patients improve after two to four weeks of medication. Patients may have persistent fatigue and achiness even after treatment, but they generally recover completely within six months. In more advanced cases, intravenous antibiotics may be necessary.

## SELF-CHECKS ARE VITAL

Because it takes 24 to 48 hours for a feeding tick to transmit the infection, you should examine yourself, your children, and your pets for ticks while you are still outside and soon after returning indoors.

If you find a tick, use a pair of tweezers to remove it. Grasp the tick as close to the skin as possible and slowly pull it straight out. After removal, apply an antiseptic such as alcohol or an antibiotic ointment. Contact your doctor if any symptoms of Lyme disease occur, especially if you know you were bitten by a tick.

## PREVENTION

To further reduce the chance of being bitten by a tick, take these precautions:

- Wear a long-sleeved shirt and hat for added protection. Ticks don't always climb up from your feet; they can also drop out of trees into your hair or upper body.
- Wear light-colored clothing so ticks can be easily spotted.
- Tuck pants into socks or boots and tuck shirts into pants.
- Spray insect repellent with DEET on exposed skin and clothing.
- Stay on trails when walking in the woods, and try to avoid brushing up against long grass where ticks are more likely to hide.

- Check yourself every 3–4 hours if you're outside for a prolonged period of time.
- At home:

  ◆ Keep your lawn trimmed and cut back low-lying bushes.
  ◆ Remove leaves and tall grass around your house and garden.
  ◆ Keep woodpiles neat, off the ground, and in a sunny area or under cover to keep dry.
  ◆ Remove from your garden or yard plants that attract deer.

- Check yourself and your children carefully whenever you come in from outdoors, even if you've only been out by a swimming pool.

## VACCINE NOW AVAILABLE

In December 1998, the FDA approved a new Lyme vaccine. It has been proven effective for patients between the ages of 15 and 70.

Most vaccines work by introducing a small amount of disease into the body so that antibodies will be produced to fight the disease. This vaccine takes the process one step further by producing antibodies that travel to the site of the bite. As the infected tick begins to feed, the antibodies move into the tick's body and kill off the offending germs before they can be transmitted to you. You're protected, and the tick is cured.

For optimal protection, you'll need three doses. The second shot should be given 30 days after the first, and the third shot should be administered between 1 and 12 months after the second injection.

Reaction to this initial vaccine has been mixed. It is only 80 percent effective; it does not protect against other tick-borne illnesses; and we do not know how long it remains effective. In addition, once a person has been vaccinated, it is no longer possible to test for Lyme disease, since the vaccine stimulates antibodies that mimic the presence of the disease.

Nonetheless, the development of this vaccine marks an important medical advance, and more vaccines will be on the market soon.

A vaccine for pets is also currently available.

## ONE TOP TIP TO TEACH YOUR CHILDREN

If you live in an area where there are a lot of deer ticks, teach your children to check themselves for ticks as routinely as they brush their teeth.

## HOT BUTTON

- If you live in tick territory, check yourself, your family, and your pets regularly. Detection is the only true form of protection.
- Keep asking your doctor about new developments. The vaccines are going to keep getting better and better.
- For more information about Lyme disease, call the American Lyme Disease Foundation: (800) 876-LYME.

# Rabies

Rabies is the most rapidly fatal virus known to man. Worldwide, the statistics on rabies infection are quite high, with 30,000 people a year dying of it, mainly in developing countries where dogs are not vaccinated and treatment is not available.

In this country, where vaccination and preventive injections are available, rabies is rare in humans, with no more than a few cases occurring per year. Rabies can be carried by raccoons, bats, skunks, foxes, and coyotes, as well as domesticated pets (including ferrets). From 1990 until 1998—the most recent year for which statistics are available—20 of the 27 cases diagnosed in the United States were associated with bats.

The biggest mistake people make when it comes to rabies is thinking they have to be bitten by a "ferocious" animal to contract the disease. Nothing could be further from the truth. You can get rabies from the sweet kitten living under your neighbor's back porch if it hasn't been vaccinated. The kitten doesn't even have to bite you. Like AIDS, rabies can be transmitted by coming in contact with any body fluid—urine, semen, blood, saliva, tears, pus, etc.

## ABOUT RABIES

Rabies is one of the few viruses that can be transferred from animals to humans. It attacks the central nervous system, the brain and spinal column. For humans the incubation period is about 21 to 120 days. It is always fatal if not treated, and from initial infection to death is only four to six weeks.

The illness begins with irritation at the site of the wound, accompanied by depression and anxiety. As the disease progresses, nervousness and terror may be accompanied by excessive thirst, and a general feeling of choking or strangulation. Death results from cardiac or respiratory failure.

There are two forms of rabies: "Furious" rabies, which affects the brain and causes the animal to become aggressive or excitable (the "mad dog" of rabies fame); and "paralytic" or "dumb" rabies, which mainly affects the spinal cord and causes weakness or lethargy. A wild animal acting unusually tame may be demonstrating early warning signs of rabies.

## TREATMENT

Louis Pasteur created the first rabies vaccine in 1885, using live rabies virus. This early vaccine sometimes caused serious, even fatal reactions, but it was a start and led to the vaccines we use today.

When people talk of the shots for rabies, most are thinking of a treatment that is no longer used. It involved 21 painful shots in the abdomen, and was quite an unpleasant experience. Today most shots are given intramuscularly, usually in the shoulder, and treatment involves only five shots over a period of time.

## PREVENTION

Experts agree that preventing rabies in people depends on controlling rabies in animals. But until there is a solution for controlling it in wildlife and 100 percent compliance in owners vaccinating their pets, rabies will continue to be an infectious disease that we'll have to keep in the back of our minds. Here are measures you can take to reduce your risk:

- Keep pet vaccinations up-to-date and observe leash laws.
- Don't leave your dog chained alone in the yard. If it is attacked by a rabid animal, it can't escape, and you won't know what has happened.
- Don't make your house or yard attractive to wild animals. Feed your pet indoors and keep garbage cans closed tightly.
- Seal basement, porch, and attic openings and cap chimneys with screens. Be sure to use window screens to prevent bats from getting into the house. (Also see "Bats" for additional information.)
- No matter how adorable they are, avoid contact with wild or unfamiliar animals. One family took in a baby skunk whose mother had been killed. When they contacted ani-

mal authorities about what to do with it, they were informed that the skunk could be rabid, and it had to be killed to be tested.

- Don't touch a wild animal even if it's dead. While rabies is a temperature-sensitive virus and needs a warm-bodied host in order to live, the disease can still be communicated for about an hour after the host has died.
- Report strays or animals that are acting strangely.
- Keep heavy work gloves handy in case you're ever faced with an emergency.

## IF YOU ENCOUNTER A WILD ANIMAL

- If the animal approaches you, back away slowly, facing the animal. Never turn your back on a rabid animal. Get inside. Keep children and pets indoors with you.
- Let the animal go away on its own. Don't throw things at it or make loud noises.
- Check with the police or your county's health authority. Depending on the animal and what it's doing, local professionals may be willing to remove the animal for you. (An animal that is threatening people or pets will be considered a public nuisance in most cases.)
- If the police cannot help you, call a nuisance wildlife control officer, who will come and remove the animal for a fee.
- If a seemingly rabid animal crosses your deck or patio, keep people and pets indoors. After it is clearly gone, cover up with gloves, long-sleeved shirt and pants, and hose down the area with your garden hose, using cold water. Leave the area alone overnight, and the virus should be dead by morning.
- If your pet is exposed to an animal that might be rabid:

  ◆ Wear gloves to handle your pet. Saliva from the rabid animal may be on your pet's fur.

- Isolate your pet from other animals and people for several hours.
- Call your veterinarian. Vaccinated pets will need a rabies booster shot within 5 days of the attack.
- Call the county health authority if you need additional advice. If your pet isn't vaccinated, it must be quarantined for six months or humanely destroyed.

## WHAT TO DO IF BITTEN BY A WILD ANIMAL

- Immediately wash the wound with lots of soap and running water.
- In all likelihood, you shouldn't try to capture the animal yourself; call the police or an animal control specialist and try to get help. If it can be tested and does not have rabies, you won't have to go through the series of preventive shots.
- Get medical attention right away. If the animal is rabid, it's important to start treatment before symptoms appear. Go to your family doctor or the nearest emergency room.
- Call your county health authority.

## WHAT TO DO IF BITTEN BY A CAT OR DOG

- Immediately wash the wound with lots of soap and running water.
- Obtain the pet owner's name, address, and telephone number. Find out if the animal has a current rabies vaccination and write down the rabies tag number.
- Get medical attention. Go to your family doctor or an emergency room. Even if the pet isn't rabid, you may need a tetanus shot or to be put on an antibiotic.

## REPORTING ANY BITES

- When you report the incident to a doctor or the county health authority, that person will need to know:

  - if it was a pet, whether it wore a collar, tags, and where it lives.
  - how the bite occurred.
  - whether the animal has been seen in the area before and in what direction it was traveling.

## TWO TOP TIPS TO TEACH CHILDREN ABOUT RABIES

1. Stay away from wild animals.
2. Don't ever pet a dog or cat you don't know unless there is an owner with it. Then ask permission.

## HOT BUTTON

- Vaccinate all pets, and keep shots up-to-date.
- Check with your vet if you have any concern about whether or not your pet has come in contact with a bat or a wild animal.

# Chapter 11

# Weather-Related Disasters

## Introduction

Everyone enjoys talking about the weather, but this is especially true at the National Oceanic and Atmospheric Administration, where there are some exciting new developments in making seasonal forecasts. For the first time, the NOAA is able to lay out a reasonably accurate look at hurricane season, and day-to-day predictions are becoming more exact as well. Ten years ago, the five-day forecast wasn't exactly a "best guess," but it was close to it. Today, thanks to new technology, including Doppler radar and special weather satellites, the National Weather Service can predict one- and two-day forecasts with 90 percent accuracy.

Why is this important? You'd like to know that it's going to rain on Saturday, but not being prepared is usually more an inconvenience than a disaster.

But think of the times when the weather is actually life-threatening: One need only read about Midwest tornadoes or think of the recent fatal crash of an airliner that landed during a level six thunderstorm (the most severe) to realize that the more we know, the safer we can be.

We will always need to be respectful of the weather. With the increased potential for catastrophic property damage and loss of life along the coasts, it has become even more important for federal, state, and local governments and businesses and individuals to pay attention and take precautions whenever possible.

This section is filled with lots of weather-related specifics, but here is some general information you should know:

A National Weather Service Watch is a message indicating that conditions favor the occurrence of a certain type of hazardous weather. For example, a severe thunderstorm watch means that a severe thunderstorm is expected in the next six hours within an area approximately 120–150 miles wide and 300–400 miles long (36,000–60,000 square miles). These watches are issued by the NWS Storm Prediction Center. Local NWS forecast offices issue other watches (flash flood, winter weather, etc.) 12–36 hours in advance of a possible hazardous-weather or flooding event. Each local forecast office usually covers a state or a portion of a state.

An NWS Warning indicates that a hazardous event is occurring or is imminent in about 30 minutes to an hour. Local NWS forecast offices issue warnings on a county-by-county basis.

Though watches are not as high status as warnings, they are more important than people realize. If your area is on the front edge of the storm, you may be the first to learn that this particular weather condition now merits a full warning.

There are some specific things you can do to protect yourself in most hazardous weather:

- Pay attention to the weather. Listen to warnings or bulletins.
- If you're planning a car trip, a camping trip, or any kind of travel, listen to the weather so that you'll be forewarned of what to expect. If you're vacationing in Florida in August, there's always the possibility you might experience a hurricane, for example, so you might refresh your memory about precautions to take before you go.
- Periodically remind your community of the importance of maintaining its emergency warning systems.

- Read the information in this section and take the precautions that are appropriate for your area.

## WHAT IS EL NIÑO AND LA NIÑA ANYWAY?

Since El Niño has been blamed for almost all the weather we've had in recent years, it seems important to explain it.

El Niño refers to a change in the Pacific trade winds. About once every four to seven years, the trade winds calm or reverse, and the warm water that usually travels toward the western coasts of the South Pacific instead travels backward, toward the eastern coasts of the Pacific, where the water is cool and nutrient-rich. Rainfall follows the warm water east, causing flooding in South America, and leaving the western countries prone to drought. The rise in warm, humid air then affects the jet stream, pushing it off course and affecting the global atmospheric circulation, changing weather patterns all over the world. The name El Niño, referring to the Christ child, was chosen because the warm waters usually start around Christmas near Peru.

La Niña refers to cooler-than-average sea-surface temperatures across the central and eastern tropical Pacific Ocean, which historically have contributed to a greater number of hurricanes in the Atlantic during a given season.

While there is nothing threatening about "El Niño" or "La Niña" in and of themselves, the changes they bring about can create dangerous situations; they set off some of the severe forms of weather that are described next.

# Avalanches*

Like an earthquake that occurs in a distant, uninhabited area, the avalanche that falls unnoticed in an unpopulated area is a natural phenomenon that holds no hazard to people if no one is around to be hurt by it. However, as more and more people participate in winter sports, pushing the boundaries for skiing, snowboarding, snowshoeing, and snowmobiles, the chances for sports participants to trigger or get caught in these formerly unnoticed avalanches increases.

Largely because of a rapid increase in the number of backcountry skiers, snowboarders and snowmobilers, the average count of Americans killed by avalanches has gone up, rising from 7 a year in the 1970s to 24 a year in the 1990s. Between 1950 and the winter of 1998–99, 573 people are known to have died in 429 separate snow avalanches in the United States alone. Of these 573, four out of five, or 80 percent were recreationists. A majority of the victims triggered the avalanches that killed them.

Only recently the European Alps experienced a devastating avalanche season. Some of the highest snowfalls in half a century set off vast snowslides and killed dozens of people, catching many of them in houses built on sites where avalanches are most likely to occur. Those who weren't hurt in the actual avalanche were trapped by the snow and couldn't leave the area. Witnesses described it as "happening in a split second": It turned dark and then the area was engulfed in snow.

The same scenes could one day be repeated in snowy climates in the United States where the populations of some mountain counties are expected to double over the next 25 years with more and more people building homes in avalanche territory.

No one could be more aware of the "avalanche problem" than the tourist industry, and many steps are being taken to avoid injuries. Most mountain states work hard to keep the number of

---

* An avalanche usually consists of snow and ice; a landslide is made up of rocks, soil, mud, and debris, and a lahar is a landslide containing lava that results from a volcanic eruption.

deaths down by aggressive education programs, which generally involve sending out e-mail alerts, running classes, broadcasting daily messages on mountain radio stations, holding safety classes for vacationers, and fielding incoming telephone queries about avalanches.

Learning about avalanches and how to survive them is taking on new importance for those who spend time in snow country. One need only consider that Alex Lowe, a 40-year-old mountaineer described by colleagues as "the best climber of his time," lost his life in 1999 to an avalanche to understand the seriousness of learning everything you can about these phenomena.

## WHAT HAPPENS IN AN AVALANCHE?

There are several kinds of avalanches, among them:

The *loose snow* avalanche—the cartoon-style avalanche—occurs when loose snow starts rolling downhill, becoming a bigger and bigger snowball.

In a *slab* avalanche, the top layer of snow begins to slide, the way a large cookie sheet would slide down a hill. This snow can travel as fast as 80–100 miles per hour, though a wet, full-depth slab might travel much more slowly, at a "turtle-like" 10–15 miles per hour.

Sometimes gravity will pull down an overhanging chunk of snow, resulting in a *cornice collapse*, which often triggers yet another avalanche below it.

No matter what the style, an avalanche is impressive.

Most avalanches occur soon after a heavy snowstorm. They are not acts of God; they happen because of the interaction of three variables—terrain, weather, and snowpack—but the most frequent trigger in avalanche accidents is the weight of a person passing through an avalanche-prone area. The avalanche can bury an entire village or a single skier. People sometimes die as a result of the blow from the snow (with wet snow, it can be like being plowed over by a wall of concrete); other times, they may survive for a time, but succumb to suffocation if they aren't found quickly. Still others die from exposure to the cold or shock.

Time is of the essence in locating victims. There is over a 90 percent probability of survival if the person is found in the first 15 minutes, but it drops to less than 50 percent within a half hour. For that reason, it is vital that backcountry travelers carry rescue tools with them and know how to use them. There is no time to go for help.

## DRESSING FOR THE OCCASION

In addition to worrying about avalanches, winter athletes need to consider the risk of frostbite and hypothermia. (See "Winter Storms.")

- Dress in layers of clothing that are designed for winter sports. Wool, Gortex, and Lycra are excellent materials because they allow the sweat to evaporate while still protecting against the cold.
- Be sure to wear something around your head and neck to prevent excessive heat loss. A parka that comes up around your head or a face mask will also protect you against the wind.
- Mittens are preferable to gloves because they allow the fingers to warm each other.

## MANAGING FROSTBITE

Surface frostbite can happen anytime the temperature falls below freezing. When you're participating in outdoor sports, you want to recognize and deal with surface frostbite to lessen the risk of permanent damage from deep frostbite. Symptoms of early frostbite involve numbness and a white or pale look to the skin. Your partner may notice a white spot on your cheek or face, or you may notice it on your hands.

- Here's how to warm up various body parts:

  - ◆ Fingers: Place the affected parts inside your parka, in your own armpits, or against the skin; leave them there until they are warm again.
  - ◆ Toes: You'll need to get them out of your boots, so take a break and go inside to warm up. Place your bare feet against skin (or something warm) until thawed.
  - ◆ Cheeks, nose, ears, chin: Thaw them with a warm hand or other warm (not hot) object, or pull the parka hood snugly around your face until the affected area is warm and pink.

- Protect the frozen area from further exposure because it will freeze again more easily than other skin.
- Deep frostbite is a major injury. If surface frostbite is getting the best of you, it's time to call it a day and go inside.

## A "MUST HAVE" AND A "MUST DO" FOR AVALANCHE COUNTRY

- When planning a trip into what could be avalanche territory, purchase an avalanche rescue beacon at your local sporting goods store and wear it at all times. These beacons are small electronic devices capable of transmitting and receiving a signal within a range of approximately 50 to 150 feet. For the duration of a trip, each member of the group should wear their beacon on their body (tucked inside their clothes) in "transmit" mode. Should a member of the group become buried, the others should switch their beacon to "receive" mode and perform an orderly search. It will increase your chances of being found, assuming your partner has one, too, and knows how to use it. People wearing beacons have been killed by avalanches, even when dug out quickly. If you or members of your party aren't proficient at using the beacon to search, the value of wearing the device is diminished.

- In addition, you should also have with you an avalanche probe and shovel as well as an inclinometer so that you can measure slope angles (an angle of anywhere from 25–60 degrees is capable of having an avalanche).
- Some ski areas offer classes in which you can learn more about avoiding avalanches. It's worth your time. Even expert skiers and mountaineers can get caught if they aren't paying attention (Go on the Internet and look at "avalanche accident" reports, and you'll realize how important prevention is. Good Web sites to check are Avalanche.org and CSAC.org).

## AVOIDING AN AVALANCHE

- You don't have to be in remote territory to be in avalanche country. They happen in well-traveled areas as well.
- When traveling in avalanche country, you must be aware of the possibility of an avalanche at any time. Many people get caught at the end of the day when they probably become less watchful.
- If you are hiking, skiing, climbing, or camping in snowy mountain areas, read and obey all avalanche warnings.
- Avoid avalanche terrain. Slope steepness, previous avalanche activity, open bowls, and narrow gullies pose the greatest danger. Also be watchful of slopes where the wind may have led to a heavier-than-usual buildup of snow. Your safest path will be across broad ridges.
- If traveling along a ridge, stay off cornices (overhanging deposits of windblown snow); cornice failures are a common type of avalanche accident.

- Do not ever assume an area is safe because someone else traveled it, or because it's a good summer trail. During the winter, every move you make through this type of territory needs to be evaluated.
- Always follow weather reports before venturing out.

## WHAT TO DO IF CAUGHT:

- Shout to your companions the second you know what is happening. If they have a visual sighting of where you are, it will help speed the rescue.
- Toss away from you anything that you're holding—ski poles, stick, etc.
- Grab something stable to hold on to if you can—a tree or rock, for example.
- If you're downhill from a coming avalanche, try to get behind a rock or tree. Cover your head.
- Try to stay on your feet, and keep fighting.
- As the snow comes down on you, take a breath and bring your arm up to try to cover your nose and mouth. (Keep your mouth closed throughout.)
- If you're swept away, try using a swimming motion with your arms to stay on top of the snow, and keep your mouth closed. Fight for air space around your face and chest.
- If there are rocks mixed in with the snow, roll into a ball.
- The most important thing is to keep moving upward if you can.
- As the avalanche loses momentum and the snow starts to settle, use all your strength to try to thrust yourself above the snow surface, and use your arm to try to create an air space in front of your face.
- Try to take note of where other members of your party were when you last saw them. It may help in assuring their survival.

- If you've been flipped around and are disoriented, spit. Start trying to work your way up in the opposite direction that your spit fell.
- Though this is easier said than done, try to keep calm. Your hope for survival depends on conserving oxygen so that you have enough air to breathe until rescuers arrive.

## RESCUE

As in a water rescue for a drowning victim, there is an exceedingly narrow window of time for an avalanche rescue, so your best defense is not to get caught in the first place. However, if someone in your party is caught, your first task is to try to note where they were last seen. Next, start looking for clues as to where the person may be buried; these clues can be anything from the sighting of a ski tip to blood on the snow. Search quickly and thoroughly. You are the victim's prime hope.

## ONE TOP TIP TO TEACH CHILDREN ABOUT AVALANCHES

Stress the importance of taking avalanche warnings seriously, and if you have children who are mountain climbers or skiers, make sure they become experts at recognizing avalanche warning signs. Not knowing the risks in avalanche country may mean disaster for your child.

## HOT BUTTON

- If you are going to participate in backcountry winter sports, develop avalanche awareness skills. Take a class, read about avalanches, and seek the advice of others.

- Buy and wear a transmitter when in backcountry.
- If caught, try to fight to get toward the surface.

# Earthquakes

When talk turns to earthquakes, we quite naturally think of California, the scene of the famous 1906 San Francisco earthquake and the state where the San Andreas fault lies.

What we tend to ignore are the facts. There are 41 states and territories in the United States at moderate to high risk for earthquakes, and no region of the country is immune:

- Alaska experiences the greatest number of large earthquakes—most located in uninhabited areas. One of the most powerful occurred near Anchorage in 1964 and measured 9.2 on the Richter scale. In some places the ground lifted 30 feet, and the earthquake set off a tsunami that killed 122 people.
- The strongest earthquakes felt in the United States occurred along the New Madrid Fault in Missouri, where a three-month-long series of quakes from 1811 to 1812 included three quakes larger than a magnitude of 8 on the Richter scale. These earthquakes were felt over the entire Eastern United States with Missouri, Tennessee, Kentucky, Indiana, Illinois, Ohio, Alabama, Arkansas, and Louisiana experiencing the strongest ground shaking.

Part of our thinking about California is correct; the state does experience the most frequent, damaging earthquakes. The state's San Andreas fault is almost an identical twin to the North Anatolian fault that produced the magnitude 7.4 earthquake near Ismit, Turkey, in 1999, killing more than 15,000 with uncounted numbers buried in the rubble. In addition, scientists have for the first time confirmed that downtown L.A. is situated on what is known as a blind thrust fault, a type of fault capable of producing a devastating earthquake. (In a quake caused by a thrust fault, the blocks of earth move diagonally, almost vertically. In a strike-slip fault like the San Andreas, the opposing earth plates slide past each other horizontally.)

Like all natural disasters, the seriousness of an earthquake is as dependent on the population of the region as it is on the magnitude of the actual disaster. An earthquake of 8 or 9 on the Richter scale that occurs in a deserted area would not be viewed as seriously as would one that measures a 5 or 6 but occurs in a major city. Time of day also makes a big difference. If most people are at home and asleep, fewer people will be hurt than if it's midday and people are in office buildings, on freeways, and otherwise moving about outdoors.

What we do know is that earthquakes are going to continue to shake our world, and the only questions are "where" and "when." The most intelligent option is to learn what to do should a tremor begin.

## ABOUT EARTHQUAKES

The cause of an earthquake is relatively easy to understand when you recall that the earth is made up of plates of rocks that shift and move. Generally the movement is gradual, but sometimes the plates become locked together. As when any two forces are shoved together, at some point something's got to give. When enough pressure accumulates, the plates break free, setting off an earthquake.

As we learn through any news coverage of major earthquakes, a strong one can collapse buildings and bridges, disrupt gas, electric, and phone service, and sometimes trigger landslides, avalanches, flash floods, fires, and huge destructive ocean waves (tsunamis).

Often, however, the major devastation from an earthquake occurs from the events it spawns: the 1906 earthquake in San Francisco was serious, but it was the devastation of three days of fires that caused the most serious damage. Because of broken water mains, it was impossible to fight the fires. Twenty-eight thousand buildings were destroyed; three hundred thousand people were left homeless, and the death toll was approximately 700.

While the shaking of the earth is frightening, it is seldom the direct cause of death or injury. Building collapses, flying glass, and falling objects are generally the cause of earthquake-related injuries. This is extremely instructive in making adequate preparations. You will likely be able to withstand the earth tremor; what you need to focus on is creating an environment that diminishes hazards from other risk factors such as falling objects.

## HOW EARTHQUAKES ARE MEASURED

Seismographs located all over the world measure the shaking of the earth. The measure of earthquakes we all hear about is the Richter scale. In 1935 Dr. Charles Richter, a geologist at the California Institute of Technology, proposed using his method, which is actually a mathematical scale measuring the magnitude of ground movement.

Richter scale measurements run from zero to more than 9, and each number on the scale is 10 times greater than the one before it. Therefore, an earthquake measuring 6 on the Richter scale is 10 times stronger than an earthquake measuring 5 and 100 times stronger than one measuring 4. Earthquakes that register below 4 on the Richter scale are considered minor. Those of 4 or more are considered major.

Here's a general idea of what Richter scale measurements might mean to you if you were to experience an earthquake:

**0–2:** Earthquake is recorded by instruments, but is not felt by people.
**2–3:** Earthquake is felt slightly by a few people.
**3–4:** People feel tremors. Hanging objects like ceiling lights swing.

**4–5:** Earthquake causes some damage; walls crack; dishes and windows may break.

**5–6:** Furniture moves; earthquake seriously damages weak buildings.

**6–7:** Furniture may overturn; strong buildings are damaged; walls and buildings may collapse.

**7–8:** Many buildings are destroyed; underground pipes break; wide cracks appear in the ground.

**Above 8:** Total devastation, including buildings and bridges; ground wavy.

Like the waves created by a pebble tossed into water, the ripples of an earthquake weaken as they get farther and farther from the epicenter of the quake. Because the earthquake will affect all areas differently and it's impossible to measure each spot where an earthquake is felt, the measurement of any earthquake is usually gathered from at least two different seismographs and a range of the magnitude is presented, such as from a low of 7.6 to a high of 8.5.

## TO BEGIN

You may already know your neighborhood is prone to earthquakes, but if you're unsure, call your local buildings department or the local Emergency Management office.

Also talk to your insurance agent. Different parts of the country have different requirements for earthquake protection. Study the locations of active faults in your area. If you are at risk, consider purchasing earthquake insurance.

## ELIMINATING HAZARDS AT HOME

- Upgrade your home to meet current seismic building standards and safe land use codes. If you're buying a new home, look for one that meets building codes and standards and one that is built on rock, not on landfill, soil, or sediment, substances that are more likely to shift during an earthquake.

- Consider having your building evaluated by a professional structural design engineer. Ask about home repair and strengthening tips for exterior features such as porches, front and back decks, sliding glass doors, canopies, carports, and garage doors.
- Ask if your home is bolted to its foundation. These homes are less likely to be severely damaged during earthquakes.
- Repair any deep cracks in ceilings or foundations. Get expert advice if there are signs of structural defects. Earthquakes can turn cracks into ruptures and make smaller problems bigger.
- Chimneys are one of the first structures to topple in a quake, so brace it and reinforce the ceiling in that area.
- Install flexible pipe fittings to avoid gas or water leaks. Flexible fittings are less likely to break.
- Anchor all your appliances. If a heavy appliance shifts, it may rupture the gas or electric line, causing serious problems.
- Strap the water heater to wall studs. This may be your best source of drinkable water after an earthquake, so try to protect it from damage.
- Bolt bookcases, china cabinets, and other tall furniture to wall studs.
- Install strong latches on cupboards.
- Within cabinets, move large or heavy objects and fragile items to lower shelves. This will reduce your risk of being injured from a toppled statue or vase.
- Do the same in the kitchen by putting breakable items such as bottled food, glassware, and china in low closed cabinets with latches to help keep items inside.
- Store weed killers, pesticides, and flammable products securely in closed cabinets with latches. These will be less

likely to create a hazardous situation if they are stored in lower, confined locations.

- Brace overhead light fixtures. Understandably, these are the most common items to fall and cause damage or injury.
- Don't place beds under windows.
- Hang heavy items such as pictures and mirrors away from beds, couches, and anywhere people sit.
- Secure items that might fall (TV, books, computers, etc.).

## FAMILY EARTHQUAKE DRILLS

In conjunction with securing the house, you need to decide with the family what each of you will do in case of an earthquake. If all family members are at home:

- If you're in bed, stay there. You're not going to be able to get to a safe place quickly enough, and so long as you don't have a heavy painting or mirror on the wall above your bed, or a filled bookcase to one side of you, then you're about as safe as can be. Teach family members to hold on and use their pillows to protect their heads. (If you're in an area that frequently suffers earthquakes, you might want to stick a sturdy pair of shoes underneath each person's bed. One of the major injuries after an earthquake are cuts to the feet from stepping on broken glass.)
- Walk through the household with family members and choose a safe place in each room of your home. A "safe spot" is a place where you can crawl under something so that you won't be hit by falling objects. A doorway can be fine, but under a sturdy table or desk is even better, particularly if it's closer to where you are at the time a tremor starts. Remember, the fewer steps you have to take, the safer you will be.
- As you select spots, avoid anything near windows, mirrors, or picture frames unless you can be very well covered. Also

avoid fireplaces and around chimneys. Cabinets, refrigerators, and bookcases may topple so you don't want to be near them, either.

- In rooms like the kitchen or family room, you'll need to locate several safe spots. If the entire family is watching television together in the family room, point out four or five places that would be good—that way you're not all trying to crouch under one small-ish table.
- Practice in each room. Teach the whole family to clamber under a sturdy table or desk and to *drop, get under cover, and hold on*. Protect eyes by pressing your face against your arm.
- Conduct drills at least twice a year.
- As you practice with the family, remind them of a few pieces of information they should know in case of any emergency:

  - where you keep the first aid, disaster supplies, and evacuation kit
  - where the fire extinguishers are located (older kids should be taught how to use them)
  - who your out-of-area emergency contact is.

## PLANNING FOR TIMES WHEN YOU'RE NOT ALL TOGETHER

- Find out what the earthquake disaster plans are for your place of employment and children's schools.
- Make it very clear that a parent will come and get your children as soon as possible. They should stay where they are until you arrive. (Los Angeles natives frequently recommend limiting your search for a nursery school to places near your home or office that you could walk to in an emergency.)

## EARTHQUAKE SUPPLIES FOR THE CAR

In addition to the emergency supplies you already have in your trunk, people who live in earthquake-prone areas need to add the following items:

- A pair of sturdy shoes to protect your feet.
- An old set of clothing (long pants and a shirt with long sleeves). Protective clothing will make it easier to get around after an earthquake.
- A supply of water. You don't know how long it will be before you'll get to a place where you'll be able to find clean water.
- Be sure you have a flashlight with extra batteries.

## WHAT TO DO WHEN SHAKING BEGINS

- DROP, COVER, and HOLD ON: Drop under a sturdy desk or table, hold on, and protect your eyes by pressing your face against your arm. If there is no table or desk nearby, sit on the floor against an interior wall away from windows, book-cases, or tall furniture that could fall on you.
- Stay indoors until the shaking stops and you're sure it's safe to exit. When you do leave a building, move quickly away from it. Many fatalities occur when people run outside of buildings only to be killed by falling debris.

## IF YOU'RE IN AN OFFICE BUILDING OR A STORE

- Move away from windows.
- Crouch under a desk, bench, or table.
- Avoid the elevator.
- Be prepared for the fact that fire alarms and sprinklers are likely to go off.

## IF YOU'RE OUTDOORS

- If you're outdoors, find a clear spot away from buildings, trees, and power lines. Drop to the ground.
- If you're near buildings, don't run to a doorway. In all likelihood, things will shake off the building, and if you're running toward it, you're in great danger of being hit by something. If you are in a mountainous area or near unstable slopes or cliffs, be alert for falling rocks and other debris that could be loosened to create a landslide.
- If you're near the ocean, a lake, or a river, move to higher ground immediately. A tsunami is a possibility, but more important, the water is almost certainly going to rise somewhat (like water sloshing in a bathtub), and you can't predict how much.

## IF YOU'RE DRIVING

The shaking of an earthquake will feel the way it does when your car tire goes flat.

- Pull to a clear location, stop and stay in the car with your seat belt fastened until the shaking has stopped. Trees, power lines, poles, street signs, and other overhead items may fall during an earthquake. Stopping the vehicle will reduce your risk. Once the shaking stops, avoid bridges or ramps that may have been damaged.
- If you're on a bridge or overpass at the time of an earthquake, keep moving to a part of the road that is on solid ground if you can. Then pull over and stop. Most bridges and overpasses (especially in California) have been built to withstand earthquakes. However, many people have vivid memories of the I-880 bridge and Bay Bridge, which partially collapsed during the Loma Prieta earthquake in 1989. What wasn't shown on the evening news, however, were the

hundreds of other bridges that did not collapse during the same quake.

## THE AFTERMATH

- Wait in your safe place until after the shaking stops and then see if you are hurt. You'll be better prepared to help others if you take care of yourself first.
- Check others for injuries. Give first aid for serious injuries.
- If you're at home or with your car, protect yourself from further danger by putting on long pants, a long-sleeved shirt, sturdy shoes, and work gloves. When you begin to move, be careful and watch for fallen or broken items.
- Expect aftershocks. These are smaller earthquakes that follow the main shock and can cause further damage to weakened buildings. Each time you feel one, DROP, COVER, and HOLD ON. Unfortunately, they are as unpredictable as the earthquake itself and can occur in the first hours, days, weeks, or even months after a quake. Never be complacent. Be aware that some earthquakes are actually foreshocks, and an even larger earthquake may follow.
- If the house seems unsafe, get everyone outside. If you are in a multistory building, use stairs not the elevator.
- Fire is the most common earthquake-related hazard. Look for and extinguish small fires, and eliminate fire hazards.
- Use battery-powered lighting. Don't use candles at all; they increase the risk of fire. Don't under any circumstances smoke in a damaged building.
- Turn off the gas if you smell gas. A gas leak can be deadly. Only a professional should turn the gas back on. Explosions have caused injury and death when homeowners have tried to turn on the gas themselves, so only turn it off if there is a leak or if local officials advise you to do so. In an area crisis, it might be weeks or months before professionals can turn it back on for you.

- Examine walls, floors, doors, and around the chimneys to make sure the building is safe and nothing is about to collapse. Look, too, at pipes. If they are damaged, contact a plumber and the water company, and don't use the water. If you don't have bottled water, get water from an undamaged water heater or by melting previously made ice cubes.
- Once you've determined your home is safe, take pictures for the insurance company before you start to clean up.
- Open closet and cabinet doors cautiously. Contents may have shifted and might fall.
- Clean up spilled medicines, bleaches, gas, or other flammable liquids right away to avoid the hazard of a chemical emergency.
- Use the telephone only to report life-threatening emergencies.
- Outside, stay away from buildings, trees, streetlights, and power lines. Many injuries occur within 10 feet of the entrance to buildings, since bricks, roofing, and other materials may fall.

## YOUR PETS

Since earthquakes come without warning, it is difficult to safeguard your pet beforehand. However, now that the initial quake has come, keep your pet with you or crate it so that it will feel more secure and avoid further injury. Watch your animal closely. Some become aggressive or defensive out of fear.

## AS A FAMILY

- Stay together. If you are separated, activate the emergency communication plan.

## TWO IMPORTANT TIPS TO TEACH YOUR CHILDREN ABOUT EARTHQUAKES

1. Practice DROP, COVER, and HOLD ON with them often enough that it becomes automatic.
2. Explain the family emergency plans to them. Little ones should be told to wait wherever they are, and no matter what, you will come to get them. Older children should be reminded to check in with the out-of-area emergency contact. If you can't get to your daughter's middle school quickly, it will be reassuring to call Aunt Mabel and learn that she's heard from all of you, and that you're fine, just temporarily separated.

## HOT BUTTON

- Go through your home room by room, identifying what would be particularly hazardous in an earthquake. Then make needed changes.
- Work out an earthquake plan with the family, and practice it at least twice a year.
- Remember, the less distance you have to move to get to a safe place, the more likely you are to avoid sustaining injury.

# Extreme Heat: The Stealth Health Threat

Perhaps because we associate many pleasant activities like swimming and the beach with warm weather, we let heat-related illnesses sneak up on us without realizing how dangerous hot temperatures can be.

When it comes to assessing deaths due to natural hazards, only the cold of winter—not lightning, hurricanes, tornadoes, floods, or earthquakes—takes a greater toll.

In this country an average of 175 people die each year from excessive heat. (This figure doesn't take into account the deaths of those whose conditions worsen and bring on death due to extreme temperatures.) During a bad year, many more people can die due to extreme heat. According to National Oceanic and Atmospheric Administration (NOAA) statistics, over 1,000 people died in U.S. heat waves in 1995, a year when temperatures were particularly hot. In the disastrous heat wave of 1980, more than 1,250 people died.

Reports by the Centers for Disease Control and Prevention show that even people who shouldn't die from heat sometimes do, simply because it gets "too darn hot." In July of 1996 the temperature in Dallas County, Texas, ranged from 101°–106° Fahrenheit (38.3°–41.1° Celsius). The maximum daily heat index (the number derived by factoring in both heat and humidity) ranged from 105°F (40.6°C) to 112°F (44.4°C) for a six-day period.

One 61-year-old woman died at home in her bedroom. There was no air-conditioning. Fans were operating in the room, but the temperature was 107°F (41.7°C), and the air moved by the fan was 104°F (40.0°C). When she was discovered mid-afternoon of that day, her body temperature was 108°F (42.2°C).

During that same summer, a 52-year-old man started feeling poorly while mowing his lawn. He collapsed moments after knocking on a neighbor's back door. On arrival at the emergency room, he had a body temperature of 107.1°F (41.7°C). The outside heat index at the time he collapsed was 109°F (42.8°C).

In both cases the primary cause of death was hyperthermia.

The stealth threat from heat is real, and scientific studies point to an increase in mortality rates as the world climate continues to warm. According to the Intergovernmental Panel on Climate Change (IPCC), the number of very hot days could double in temperate regions of the United States as our climate changes.

It's important that we not only take heat as seriously as we do any other type of severe weather, but also that we teach our children to have a healthy respect for it. While we might restrain our children's activities during the winter because we worry about them being out in the cold too long, few parents keep children out of summer programs or restrict their other activities because of the heat. For this reason it's all the more important that children learn the importance of taking proper precautions.

The best defense against heat-related illness is prevention. This fact was proven recently when heat-related deaths were actually down during the heat wave that blanketed substantial portions of the United States in 1999. This statistical improvement is attributed to programs that have been instituted in many cities and states to mitigate the effects of heat waves.

Staying cool and making simple changes in your fluid intake, activities, and clothing during hot weather can help you remain healthy and safe.

## WHAT IS CONSIDERED EXTREME HEAT?

Extreme heat is partially registered on a thermometer, but more importantly by your body.

Temperatures that hover 10 degrees or more above the average high temperature for the region is the first parameter for defining "extreme heat." This means that extreme heat for someone in Alaska is different than for someone in Texas. Other parameters include heat that lasts for a prolonged period of time, and is often accompanied by high humidity, making the heat particularly uncomfortable. A heat index is a measure of the effect of both heat and humidity on the body, and television weather forecasters frequently refer to this as the "apparent temperature," because this is what the outside temperature *feels* like. (If you're in full sunshine, add 15 degrees to the reported heat index.)

## SO WHAT'S SO BAD ABOUT GETTING HOT?

When the weather in a particular region gets very hot, our bodies can overheat, causing internal organ damage and even death.

When blood is heated above 98.6 degrees, the body cools itself by varying the rate and depth of blood circulation (bringing more blood to the surface of the skin in an attempt to cool it), by losing water through the skin through sweat glands, and if a person really overheats, by panting. When the body can no longer keep itself cool or becomes dehydrated due to the effort to cool itself, the temperature of the body's inner core begins to rise and heat-related illness may develop.

Elderly people, young children, and those who are sick or overweight are more likely to be victims. Because men sweat more than women and become dehydrated more quickly, they are more susceptible to heat illness.

Studies show a significant rise in heat-related illnesses when heat lasts more than two days. People living in urban areas may be at greater risk from the effects of a prolonged heat wave. An increased health problem, especially for those with respiratory difficulties, can occur when stagnant atmospheric conditions trap pollutants in urban areas, thus adding unhealthy air to excessive hot temperatures. In addition, asphalt and concrete store heat longer, and heat is then gradually released at night. This produces significantly higher nighttime temperatures in urban areas, known as the "urban island effect."

## WARNING SIGNS OF HEAT DISORDERS

Most heat disorders occur because the victim has been overexposed to heat or has overexercised for his or her age and physical condition.

***Heat cramps:*** This may be the first sign that you're overdoing it. These painful spasms usually affect the muscles of the legs or abdomen.

***Heat exhaustion:*** Think of this as the "you better stop now" disorder. It is usually signified by heavy sweating, paleness, muscle cramps, weakness, dizziness, headache, nausea or vomiting, or fainting. The skin may be cool and moist. The pulse rate will be fast and weak, and breathing will be fast and shallow. If heat exhaustion is untreated, it may progress to heatstroke. Seek medical help if symptoms are severe or if the victim has heart problems or high blood pressure. Otherwise, get the person to a cooler spot where he or she can sit down. The person should begin trying to cool down by drinking water and if possible, applying cool compresses.

***Heat- or sunstroke:*** This is a medical emergency, and you need to find help immediately. Heatstroke is characterized by the rapid (within minutes) rise of the core body temperature to 105°F (40.6°C) or more. Early symptoms of heatstroke include dizziness, weakness, headache, clammy skin, a slow pulse, and possibly nausea. At this stage, the sufferer may only be suffering from heat exhaustion. However, if the victim does not cool off, rest, and replenish lost body fluids and salts, his condition can progress to heatstroke, evidenced by lethargy, disorientation, delirium, and eventually coma. Death can follow.

Call an ambulance right away, then do what you can to begin to bring the victim's temperature down. Emergency treatment of heatstroke involves cooling the person with a cold bath or wet sheets. If neither is available, get the person to a shady area and pour water over his clothes while awaiting the arrival of emergency personnel.

## KEEP YOUR HOME AS COOL AS POSSIBLE

- Have a good attic fan installed so that it can provide an exhaust system for blowing out the hot air that becomes trapped in attics. The cooler the attic, the cooler your home.
- If you can't afford—or don't really need—air-conditioning for the whole house, install a window unit in at least one room. This will provide relief on any very hot days.
- Good insulation and weather-stripping on doors and windows are as important in the summer as in the winter. In

the summer you want to keep the hot air out. Some people keep their storm windows in place all year round.

- Practice heat management every day. If your region of the country doesn't call for full-time air-conditioning, open the windows at night. Close the windows, put down awnings, and draw shades or draperies during the day. Particularly in regions that aren't especially humid, you can cause a noticeable effect on the household temperature by closing out hot daytime breezes and sunlight.
- If you do have an air-conditioning unit, vacuum AC filters weekly during periods of high use. The unit will be more efficient if your filters are clean.
- Fans are only helpful when the temperature is less than 90°F (32.2°C). If temperatures are higher than this and you have no other home cooling system, go to the mall, the movies, or the public library for a few hours each day during a heat wave. People who spend at least two hours per day in air-conditioning during a period of extreme heat lessen their health risks.

## ADJUSTING YOUR FOOD AND FLUID INTAKE

The body sheds heat in two primary ways: The first involves dilated blood vessels near the skin. Blood that is heated in the body core comes to the surface to cool off. The other method is by sweat production, acting like an air conditioner. When the sweat evaporates, it gives up heat, which cools the skin. The more you sweat, the more heat you lose. Adjusting your food and fluid intake helps your body work more efficiently:

- Eat lightly. Heavy meals loaded with protein increase metabolic heat production as well as water loss.
- Drink fluids. Even if you don't feel thirsty and aren't particularly active at the time, keep drinking plenty of water. Your

body needs it to keep cool. (People who have medical conditions that restrict fluid intake or who have a problem with fluid retention should consult a doctor before increasing their consumption of fluids.)

- If the temperature is still manageable and you are exercising or working while it's hot, drink two to four glasses of cool fluids each hour.
- Avoid alcohol and caffeine. Juices and sports drinks are fine. Very cold drinks can cause stomach cramps.
- People over 65 need to be particularly mindful of drinking fluids as their bodies have a reduced ability to respond to external temperature changes.
- Do not take salt tablets unless specified by a physician. Persons on salt restrictive diets should consult a physician before increasing their salt intake.

## KEEPING COOL

Your body adjusts gradually to change. Therefore, an early summer heat wave is more difficult to deal with than one later in the summer when your body is accustomed to the warm weather. When the heat index gets above 90°, all family members should:

- Dress appropriately. Lightweight, light-colored clothing reflects heat and sunlight and helps your body maintain normal temperatures.
- Don't get too much sun. In addition to the negative effects of sunburn on the skin, getting burned also makes the job of keeping the body cool that much harder. When you are out, use a sunscreen with a high SPF rating. (Also refer to "Ozone Depletion and the Sun.")
- Wear a wide-brimmed hat to help keep your head cool and to reduce the amount of sun exposure to your face.

- NEVER leave anyone in a closed, parked vehicle. Temperatures inside a parked car can reach 140–160 degrees Fahrenheit in only a few moments.
- Slow down. Avoid strenuous activities during the middle of the day, and if it remains hot, eliminate or reduce what has to be done until the weather cools.
- Postpone outdoor games and activities. Extreme heat can threaten the health of athletes, staff, and spectators of outdoor games and activities.
- Take frequent breaks if you work outdoors or in a hot factory or office.
- Use a buddy system. When working or exercising during the summer, set up a system in which you monitor someone and they do the same for you.
- If you are feeling overly tired, stop all activity, get into a cool area, and rest—especially if you become light-headed or weak.
- Avoid extreme temperature changes. When you come in from the heat, cool off gradually. A cool shower when you've just come in can result in hypothermia, particularly for elderly and very young people.

## HEAT IS BAD FOR PETS, TOO

Heatstroke is one of the summer's most frequent afflictions for animals, and one of the most lethal. You need to do what you can to help your pet stay cool:

- Walk your dog in the early morning or late evening before the heat of the day is upon you.
- If you must go out at midday, make it brief and consider the temperature of the asphalt. The pavement can be hot enough to burn the very thick flesh of the footpads.
- A dog's body is more vulnerable to heat radiating from the

road. Temperatures at two and three feet above the ground can be 20 degrees hotter than at a man's height of six feet.

- If you're out for a prolonged period, bring along water and a collapsible bowl.
- Leave your dog at home during hot weather if you might otherwise have to leave him in a parked car. Temperatures in a car can reach 160 degrees in a matter of minutes even with the windows partially open.
- Consider your dog's coat. A lighter-skinned dog will fare better with a longer coat to guard against sunburn; other dogs will do best if the coat is cut down and combed out to help release heat from the dog.
- Know the symptoms of dog heatstroke: elevated body temperature, vigorous panting, unsteady gait, depression or agitation, thick saliva, or frothing at the nose or mouth, rigid posture, vomiting, bloody diarrhea, collapsing, and signs of shock. If your dog displays any of these symptoms, call the veterinarian, and start trying to cool the body gradually with cool (not cold) water. Let the dog drink slowly if possible.

## TWO TOP TIPS TO TEACH CHILDREN ABOUT COPING WITH HEAT

1. It's important to slow down when it's really hot.
2. Drink extra water on these days, and drink even if you're not that thirsty.

## HOT BUTTON

- During a heat wave, make it a priority to be in an air-conditioned space for part of the day. Even if you can't be cool all the time, the body needs periods of cooling off in order to withstand high temperatures.

- Dress in the coolest manner possible.
- Slow down and drink plenty of fluids.

# Floods and Flash Floods

From the Yangtze River in China to the Mississippi in the United States, countries around the world have sought to tame, channel, and control the mighty force of some of our most beautiful and powerful resources—the rivers and seas. However, as surely as night follows day, overly plentiful rains fall, or restrictive material around ice floes or debris breaks free, causing the temporarily contained water to overwhelm man-made levees and dams.

When it comes to water, we can drink it, put it to work for us, travel on it, admire it, and use it for recreation; but when there's too much of it, water always wins.

Walk down almost any river or coastal town, and chances are that a resident can tell you about "the time when . . ." In places like Pueblo, Colorado, this may be a memory from eighty years ago; in places like St. Louis, it may be very recent. Your "tour guide" will point out marks on downtown buildings that indicate how high the water reached, and he'll tell you of mass chaos and post-destruction cleanup.

Floods are among the most frequent and costly of natural disasters, and most communities are vulnerable in some way. Every state has at least one dam that is considered "high hazard" by the Army Corps of Engineers, and Pennsylvania and Texas each have over 500. North Carolina's number is even higher than that. The annual average loss of lives due to floods is 95 people per year, mainly because of flash floods, and approximately 300,000 Americans are driven from their homes by floods annually.

Flooding can come at any time of year: Melting snow can combine with rain in the winter and early spring; severe thunderstorms can bring heavy rain in the spring and summer; tropical cyclones (hurricanes) can produce intense rainfall throughout the summer and fall.

## ABOUT FLASH FLOODING

Flash floods involve sudden and unpredictable surges of water, sometimes due to heavy localized rainfall, sometimes from a dam break, the release of an ice floe, a faraway storm, or as a result of another natural disaster. It does not even have to be raining for a flash flood to occur.

The moment you feel endangered, climb to higher ground. These floods often come without warning, so you may have only seconds to make what will be a life-and-death decision as to how to reach safety.

## IF YOU REMEMBER ONLY ONE THING . . .

Don't walk or drive into flooded waters. Experts say that most people simply don't understand how serious a threat to life floodwater can be. Even six inches of fast-moving floodwater can knock you off your feet, and a depth of two feet will float your car. Never try to walk, swim, or drive through swift water. If you come upon floodwaters, *stop, turn around, and go another way*.

Remember, too, that flooding can carry away entire bridges and roadways. If the roadway is flooded, you have no way of knowing if the roadbed that was there an hour ago is still there for you to drive on now.

Because roads can flood unexpectedly, people are sometimes caught in a flash flood in their cars. In this case, you cannot risk waiting to see if the car is going to be caught in a few inches or a few feet of water—you need to get out as soon as you realize the area is flooding. It used to be that windshields could be broken and windows could be rolled down manually in emergency circumstances. On today's cars, this has become harder and harder to do, so the moment you realize water is surrounding you, open the door to break the air seal or open the windows via the power controls. You'll lose the power as the engine is submerged, so time is of the essence. Get out of your seat belt as quickly as possible and help any passengers to get free. With luck, you'll still be able to wade to higher ground before more water arrives.

## GENERAL FLOOD PROTECTION MEASURES

- Determine the magnitude of the flood risk in your area. Call your community emergency management office, the National Weather Service, or your American Red Cross chapter for information.
- If you're considering building in a floodplain, talk to area building engineers first. Some communities won't give building permits for these areas. If it is permitted, take precautions and raise your furnace, electrical panel, and water heater. An undamaged water heater is often the best source of fresh water after a flood. Also ask what you are permitted to build to stop floodwaters from coming into your property. Most communities regulate the building of barriers such as levees and flood walls.
- If you're considering buying or building on waterfront property, reconsider. It's only a matter of time until the land will flood. While you might be fortunate during your tenancy, are you prepared to take the chance?
- Talk to your insurance agent. If you don't have insurance coverage, ask about the National Flood Insurance Program. If your community has adopted resolutions and ordinances that help reduce the flood hazard in your area, you may be offered lower insurance premiums. Usually there is a five-day waiting period before this type of insurance goes into effect, so you want to have coverage in place before weather forecasters start talking about the "big flood" that's coming to your area.

- Install check valves in building sewer traps to prevent flood-water from backing up into your drains. If a flood is threatening, large corks or stoppers can help plug showers, tubs, or basins.
- Seal walls in basements with waterproofing compounds to avoid seepage through cracks.
- Talk to a construction professional about additional measures that should be taken, and check local building codes and ordinances for safety requirements.

## IF A FLOOD WATCH IS ISSUED FOR YOUR AREA

- Keep children and pets indoors.
- Fill the gas tank in your car and double-check your disaster supplies. Locate sleeping bags or extra blankets in case evacuation is necessary.
- Be alert to signs of flooding. If it's been raining hard for several hours or steadily for several days, start listening to the radio and be watchful as to what's happening outside.
- Listen to an NOAA weather radio and follow instructions.
- Bring outdoor belongings indoors. Even if no flooding occurs, bringing in miscellaneous items from outdoors before a storm is a good idea.

## IF YOU'RE AT HOME BUT THE CONDITIONS ARE WORSENING, OR IF A WARNING IS ISSUED

- Fill bathtubs, sinks, and plastic bottles with clean water.
- Selectively move your furniture and valuables to higher floors.
- Disconnect all electrical and gas appliances if there is time. Shut off the water main to keep contaminated water from the water heater (it may be your best source of emergency water).

## IF YOU DECIDE—OR ARE TOLD—TO EVACUATE

- The news and weather people can't be everywhere, so if you sense that your area is likely to flood sooner than they are saying, evacuate immediately. Gather family and pets and your disaster supplies, but don't worry about your belongings.
- Along with your supplies kit, take extra blankets and sleeping bags with you.
- Call your family's emergency contact person to report your plans.
- Leave early enough to avoid being marooned by flooded roads. Delaying may allow escape routes to become blocked.
- Follow the advice of those in charge of the evacuation.
- Use travel routes recommended by authorities.
- Keep your radio on for news and updates.
- Watch for flooding at bridges, viaducts, and low-lying areas.
- Be alert for thunder and lightning that may signify rain and more flooding ahead.
- If you come upon a flooded road, turn around and go away.

## THREE TOP TIPS TO TEACH CHILDREN ABOUT FLOODING

1. If you come to a flooded area, stop, turn around, and go another way. Climb to higher ground. Even six inches of water can knock you off your feet.
2. Never try to walk, swim, or play in floodwater. You may not realize how fast floodwater is moving or see holes and submerged debris.
3. Watch out for snakes in floodwater.

## AFTER A FLOOD OR A HURRICANE

- Put on sturdy shoes before leaving wherever you've waited out the storm.
- If anyone has been hurt, seek medical care.
- Check on people in the surrounding area.
- Report downed power lines right away.
- Don't enter any area until given the "okay" by safety officials, and stay out of any building that is still surrounded by water.

## IF YOUR HOME HAS BEEN FLOODED

Once you've been given permission to enter your home, take appropriate precautions:

- There may be frayed wires or a gas leak, so be very careful on entering. Don't smoke; use battery-powered lanterns or flashlights to examine the building. Check for fire hazards, gas leaks, or electrical system damage.
- Don't use gas-powered machines, generators, camping stoves, or charcoal grills indoors because fumes and carbon monoxide exhaust can be deadly.
- Photograph the damage for insurance purposes, and then start cleaning up.
- Throw away food, cosmetics and medicine that have gotten wet, as well as canned goods. Floodwaters contain sewage, chemicals, oil, and other health hazards which may have contaminated food, medicine, and cosmetics. Even canned items must be tossed because of possible interior damage from rust.
- Mold and mildew cause problems even for people who aren't terribly allergic, so toss mattresses and bedding that have been saturated, and remove wet carpets and wash down walls with disinfectant. You'll also need to remove wallboard, insulation, and wall coverings.

- Silt and mud left after the water recedes should be shoveled out then hosed away—both inside and out. The mud may contain health hazards, so get rid of it quickly and wear rubber gloves and, if possible, a face mask when cleaning.
- Pump any water out of basements and cellars gradually to avoid structural damage.
- Don't use any electrical appliance that has been wet, since there is a possibility of electric shock or fire.

## HOT BUTTON

- Don't take a chance in a flash flood. The moment you find the water is coming in your direction, get to higher ground.
- If you come to floodwaters, stop, turn around, and go another way.
- Don't try to drive on a flooded roadway. You have no idea whether the road that was there a few hours ago is still there.
- Be sure you have flood insurance through your own insurance policy or through the National Flood Insurance Program.

# Hurricanes

When one thinks of a high fatality rate connected with a natural disaster, earthquakes are likely the first thing that comes to mind. Yet in the United States it is a hurricane that holds the record for the greatest number of deaths from a natural disaster. On September 8, 1900, a powerful hurricane came ashore in Galveston, Texas, and buffeted the town with wind gusts of at least 120 miles per hour and massive flooding. Over 6000 people were killed.

While improved building techniques and new early warning

systems have greatly diminished hurricane deaths in the United States, it's foolhardy to say nothing like that could ever happen again. The danger is current, and it's very real. The advantage we gain through greater awareness is lost as larger populations settle into barrier islands and coastal areas where evacuation is difficult. What's more, experts say that 80–90 percent of those living in hurricane-prone areas have never experienced a significant storm. As a result, they lack the respect that is necessary when dealing with major weather events. Even residents of inland areas shouldn't feel complacent; they are vulnerable to strong winds, heavy rains, flooding, and hurricane-spawned tornadoes.

One problem that came to light during Hurricane Floyd in 1999 is the inadequacy of our nation's highway system in evacuating the population from large areas of the country all at once. As people in the Carolinas began to leave home, their progress was slowed by residents of Florida and Georgia who were already clogging roads going north. In addition, some families loaded two or three cars with possessions and as many family members who could drive took to the roads, making it difficult for other families to get out at all. While Federal Emergency Management personnel will be examining ways to ease the traffic crush in these situations, the lesson for private individuals is that you can't afford to wait.

When you leave, do so with one vehicle, and take along family and friends who might need a ride. In a major emergency a little consideration for one's fellowman makes sense.

Those who still aren't convinced these storms need to be taken seriously should consider the escalating potential for economic catastrophe. As more structures are built in vulnerable areas, property damage is skyrocketing. The country experienced this firsthand in 1992 when Hurricane Andrew hit Florida, causing about a million people to evacuate and approximately $30 billion in damages. To date Andrew is one of the most costly of any natural disaster.

Each year, on average, ten tropical storms, of which six become hurricanes, develop over the Atlantic, the Caribbean, or the Gulf of Mexico during hurricane season (June–November). For areas that are in hurricane pathways, the question isn't "if" they'll be hit, it's only "when," and how severely.

## THE NATURE OF A HURRICANE

Hurricanes, cyclones, and typhoons are all tropical storms with wind speeds that exceed 74 miles per hour. Different terminology is used in different areas of the world. In the Atlantic Ocean and in the eastern part of the Pacific (east of the international date line), such storms are called hurricanes. West of the international date line in the Pacific, they're called typhoons. In the Indian Ocean, those same tropical storms are cyclones. (The word cyclone is also used to define the general phenomena of a large circular atmospheric system.)

Hurricane winds blow in a large spiral around a relatively calm center known as the "eye." The eye is generally 20–30 miles wide, and the storm may have a diameter of 400 miles. A hurricane can bring torrential rains, high winds, and a storm surge as it nears land. A single hurricane can last more than two weeks over open water and can run a path across the entire length of the eastern seaboard.

High winds, flooding, and the potential for tornadoes create the greatest threats to life and property in this type of storm. Hurricane winds can top 160 miles per hour and are strong enough to uproot trees, demolish houses, and turn debris into deadly missiles. These big winds can drive ocean water up the mouths of rivers and, accompanied by torrential rains, compound the severity of inland flooding. Storm surges can create domes of ocean water 20 feet high and 50–100 miles wide; these surges can devastate entire coastal communities as they sweep ashore. The resulting currents are so powerful that they can erode the beach and move the shoreline several hundred feet inland. Most fatalities and property damage arise from this abundance of powerful water.

As with tornadoes and earthquakes, there is a method for ranking hurricanes: Categories range from 1 for weak cyclones to 5 for the most severe. Accordingly, the risk of property and crop damage, shore erosion, and danger to life increases from low for a category 1 to very high for a category 5 cyclone, where the winds can blow 200 miles per hour.

If there is a positive side to the modern hurricane situation, it is that we now get plenty of warning. While a tornado can still arrive unannounced, a hurricane spends plenty of time signaling that she's on the way. When you hear a storm is coming, listen carefully for its movements and take appropriate steps to protect yourself and your family.

## IF YOU'RE BUILDING IN A HURRICANE AREA

Construction near water should be on deep pile foundations. Many homes built on slab foundations have been destroyed, while nearby houses on pilings have survived. Building in an area of rapid erosion is a risky investment at best, but if the water views are too good to resist, check with your insurance agent about any particular recommendations he or she might make. Then make certain your contractor has had a great deal of experience in the area. You'll pay in the long run if you use the less expensive fellow whose experience has all been inland.

## GENERAL PREPARATION

- Talk to your insurance agent about your coverage. If you don't have adequate coverage, ask about the National Flood Insurance Program. (Refer to Chapter Five, "Insuring Against Disaster.")
- Check with your town to see if community personnel visit homes to discuss hurricane mitigation measures. If not, as a onetime expense, have an engineer check your home

and advise you about ways to make it more resistant to hurricanes. Ask about the garage doors and the roof—areas that are particularly vulnerable during high winds.

- Ideally, coastal homes should be elevated. If yours is not, talk to your local emergency manager about what you can do.
- Install permanent hurricane shutters. These are the best protection for windows and doors.
- If you don't have shutters, install anchors for plywood (marine plywood is best) and predrill holes in precut half-inch outdoor plywood boards so you can cover windows quickly. Don't forget to put something over glass doors. The danger to smaller windows is mainly from wind-driven debris; larger windows may be broken by wind pressure.
- Have necessary protective building supplies on hand for the season. Once there's a warning or a watch, you don't want to be standing in line at your building materials store.
- If you live in an area that's prone to flooding, also follow flood preparedness precautions. Some hurricanes drop more than 10–15 inches of rain in just a few hours.
- Have your rain gutters and downspouts cleaned. Clear drainage will help get the water away from your home.
- Make a list of what to bring inside in a storm to avoid additional hazards from blowing garbage cans, etc.
- Know your nearest safe high ground and the best access route as well as the location of the nearest shelter. Ask about streets that are most likely to flood.

## DISASTER SUPPLIES

- Check your disaster supplies at the beginning of hurricane season, and resupply as needed. Certainly start with new bottled water and food items.
- Keep a backup supply of prescription medicines on hand

during hurricanes. Stores and pharmacies may have difficulty keeping up with the demand after a storm.

## VACATIONER ALERT

Because beach areas and coastal towns are popular tourist spots, vacationers sometimes find themselves in the midst of a hurricane watch or warning. Because the area is unfamiliar to you, it's particularly important that you take safety precautions:

- Your first step in this process starts when planning your vacation. Check with the weather service to determine if you're visiting an area that is vulnerable to hurricanes. Some companies sell trip insurance that will cover various situations—including evacuation—if your trip has to be canceled. Depending on your costs, it may be worth the investment.
- When you arrive, find out the name of the county in which you're staying. Weather-related warnings and announcements are generally made by county (or parish, in Louisiana); it's important to know what information pertains to you and what doesn't.
- Pick up a local map.
- Just as you should check for fire exits in any hotel room or home rental, note evacuation routes (they'll be well marked) for the area you're visiting. Also talk to the hotel proprietor (or community members if you're renting a vacation home), about warnings (How is the community notified of a problem?) and evacuation procedures. A few moments of embarrassment about seeming "excessively concerned," will let you relax and enjoy your vacation completely.
- Keep your gas tank at least half full, and if there is no radio in your hotel room or home rental, pick up an inexpensive

transistor radio so that you'll have a way to keep abreast of the news if necessary.

## WHEN A HURRICANE WATCH (24–36 HOURS NOTICE) IS ISSUED

- Be ready to move to higher ground or shelter facilities if told to do so. High winds and flooded roads will make it hazardous during your transfer, so follow the advice of emergency personnel.
- Get gas if you have time. When there is no electricity, gas pumps won't work.
- Locate pets so that you can take them with you.
- Stockpile drinking water in clean bathtubs, sinks, plastic bottles, and cooking utilities. Your greatest need following a disaster will be water.
- Turn your refrigerator and freezer to the coldest setting. Open it only when absolutely necessary and close it quickly. This will help perishables last longer in the event of a power failure.
- Listen to the radio or television constantly, noting the hurricane's location and the expected intensity when it reaches landfall.
- Start closing the hurricane shutters or boarding up windows and doors.
- Don't bother taping your windows—a practice that used to be advised. According to the Central Florida Hurricane Center, tests have found taping to be a waste of time: "A little masking tape (or duct tape) is no protection against the flying debris in a hurricane, and the strength the tape adds is about the same as putting a piece of one-ply tissue paper over the window."
- Anchor outdoor items that can't be brought inside. Bring in loose garden tools, toys, and garbage cans. Secure things like awnings.

- Move boats on trailers close to the house and fill them with water to weigh them down. Lash the boat securely to the trailer and use tie-downs to anchor the trailer to the ground or house.
- Check mooring lines of boats in water, then leave them.

## WHEN A HURRICANE WARNING (24 HOURS OR LESS) IS ISSUED

- Mobile home residents should check the tie-downs on their home, and leave immediately.
- Use the telephone only when necessary at this point.
- If you have not yet been told to evacuate and feel it's safe to stay at home, select an interior room on the first floor away from windows, skylights, and glass doors. If the storm gets very bad, lie on the floor under a table. This offers the greatest protection from falling objects.
- If power is lost, unplug computers and appliances to reduce the "surge" when electricity is restored.
- Turn off utilities if told to do so by authorities. Usually they want you to leave gas on because a professional is required to turn it back on, but they may want water or electricity off.
- If you are without power, use flashlights for emergency lighting. Don't use candles or kerosene lanterns. Between 1984 and 1998, candle-related deaths from home fires following hurricanes were three times greater than the number of deaths related to the direct impact of the storm. Kerosene lamps require a great deal of ventilation and are not for inside use.
- Turn off propane tanks. Propane tanks may be damaged or dislodged by strong winds or water. Turning them off reduces the potential for fire.
- Pack an evacuation kit consisting of flashlights and batteries, appropriate clothing, sturdy shoes, personal essentials,

your first aid kit, and the plastic bag containing your important papers.

- Follow directions of emergency personnel.

## TRAVELING

- Stay away from floodwaters. Most flood fatalities are caused by people attempting to drive through water. The depth of the water isn't always obvious. The roadbed may be washed out under the water, and you could be stranded or trapped. Rapidly rising water may stall the engine, engulf the vehicle and its occupants, or sweep you away. Two feet of water will carry away most automobiles.

## IF YOU'RE AT HOME DURING A HURRICANE

- Stay indoors even during the lull of the "eye." The lull sometimes ends suddenly and winds can increase in seconds to a hurricane force of 74 mph or more.
- Stay away from windows and glass doors. Move furniture away from exposed doors and windows.
- Stay on the side of the house that's not taking the wind. Move as the wind moves. If you have an inside space without windows (a room or a hallway), stay there during the height of the hurricane.
- Stay in touch via television as long as you can and then switch to a battery-powered radio if the power goes out. Unexpected changes can sometimes call for last-minute relocations.
- Remain calm.

## IF YOU ARE TOLD TO EVACUATE

- Before leaving, secure your property, and if you have not already done so, turn off the electricity and main water valve and unplug appliances quickly before you leave.
- Call your designated contact regarding your whereabouts so that distant family members will know where you are.
- Don't travel farther than necessary. Roads can be jammed. Leave early so that you can travel by daylight. Dangerous winds and tides may arrive three to five hours before the hurricane.
- Wear sturdy shoes and take extras if you can.
- In addition to your disaster supplies, remember to bring:

  - clothing that can be layered
  - first aid kit, manual, prescriptions
  - baby food and diapers
  - cards and games, books
  - toiletries
  - radio and extra batteries
  - flashlight (one per person) and extra batteries
  - blankets or sleeping bags
  - ID
  - valuable papers (copies of insurance papers, passports, and other essential documents).

- Hard as it is to leave your home at times of stress, it's important that you do so. Lock up and leave.

## IF YOU EVACUATE: THE AFTERMATH

- Don't go outside until you're officially advised that the storm has passed.
- If you had to evacuate, don't go home until you're advised to do so.

- Continue listening to a local radio station to be certain that you're aware of any new developments.
- Use the recommended evacuation route and walk or drive cautiously. Debris-filled streets are dangerous. Snakes and poisonous insects will be a hazard, and washouts may weaken road and bridge structures, which could collapse under the weight of your vehicle.
- Don't go sightseeing to survey the damage. It's important to keep the roads clear for emergency personnel.
- Be careful of fallen trees, damaged buildings, flooded areas, and fallen power lines. If you see a downed power line, call the power company. Many lives are lost to electrocution.
- Never try to walk, swim, or drive through swift water. If the water is fast-moving, even water six inches deep can sweep you off your feet.

## CLEANING UP AT HOME

- For insurance purposes, photograph the damage that has occurred, and contact your insurance representative. There will be people on the scene to work closely with you after a major disaster. If your home is not livable, provide your rep with a number where you can be contacted. Plan to make temporary repairs, and do what you can to prevent the possibility of further damage from rain. (Save all receipts. The expenses may be covered by your insurance policy.)
- Remain alert for additional rainfall and flooding, even after the hurricane or tropical storm has passed.
- Examine walls, floors, doors, staircases, and windows to make sure that the building is not in danger of collapsing. Pump out a flooded basement gradually (about one-third per day) to avoid structural damage.
- Service damaged septic tanks, cesspools, pits, and leaching systems as soon as possible. Damaged sewage systems are health hazards.

- Use a stick to poke through any debris, watching for animals, particularly poisonous snakes.
- Open windows and doors to ventilate and dry the house. Pull up soggy carpet and scrub away mold and mildew with disinfectants. Allergies will almost inevitably worsen until these allergens are minimized.
- Guard against spoiled food. If the refrigerator is off for more than a few hours, you'll need to throw out most of the contents. Freezers will keep food safe for several days if the doors are kept shut, but don't refreeze food after it begins to thaw.
- Don't use tap water until you're sure it's safe. Use your emergency supply or boil water for ten minutes before drinking or until you receive official word that the water is safe.

## GUARD AGAINST FIRE

- Because of broken water mains, water pressure is often low after a storm, which can make firefighting very difficult.
- If your home was flooded, have an electrician inspect your system before turning it back on.
- Watch for fire hazards.
- Look for gas leaks. If you smell gas or hear a hissing sound, open a window and quickly leave the building. Turn off the gas using the outside main valve if you can, and call the gas company from a neighbor's home.

## THREE TOP TIPS TO TEACH CHILDREN ABOUT HURRICANES

Since there should be plenty of warning about a hurricane, your children will almost certainly be with you. Start teaching them the following so that one day they'll know it for themselves:

1. Take hurricane warnings seriously, and follow the instructions given by emergency personnel.
2. The "eye" of the hurricane is only the midpoint of the storm. Just because the weather calms down doesn't mean it's safe to go outside.
3. In the aftermath of a hurricane, children need to be careful of fast-moving water and the possibility of snakes in the debris.

## HOT BUTTON

- When a hurricane warning is issued, secure everything that you can. Leave immediately if told to do so by local officials.
- If you're at home during a hurricane (and were not told to leave), wait out the storm in an interior room to avoid the risk of being hit by blowing glass.
- If the power goes out, only use flashlights for emergency lighting.
- In the aftermath, be aware of health hazards such as unsafe water, spoiled food, and damaged electrical systems. Check each situation out one by one before assuming you can settle back into your home.

# Landslides

"Six Hikers Die in Landslide at Waterfall in Hawaii" reads a headline from *The New York Times* from May 11, 1999.

The hikers, among dozens who were exploring the Koolau Range about 30 miles north of Honolulu, certainly never thought that after stopping to enjoy the sun next to a beautiful mountain pool they might never return. Yet bad luck had it that these six died and dozens more were injured when a landslide "sent tons of boulders—some the size of compact cars—crashing down on hikers. . . ."

News stories like this remind us that nature is a force to contend with and that even when we're involved in seemingly harmless activities, we always need to keep a sharp eye out for signs of possible trouble.

## ABOUT LANDSLIDES

Landslides are a serious geologic hazard common to almost every state in the United States. It is estimated that nationally they cause 25–50 deaths annually and up to $2 billion in damages.

These "earthslides" typically follow periods of heavy rainfall or rapid snowmelt because these dynamics increase the weight of the topsoil and lubricate the underlying layers. However, wildfires can also lead to landslides because the fire strips the hill or mountainside of the vegetation that helps anchor the soil.

Some landslides move slowly and cause damage gradually; others move so rapidly that they destroy property and take lives suddenly and unexpectedly. Debris flows, also referred to as mud slides or mudflows (lahars if they are the result of a volcano) are common types of fast-moving landslides. They usually start on steep hillsides as shallow landslides, and though they generally move at about ten miles per hour, they can accelerate to speeds exceeding 35 miles per hour. (Imagine a flow of watery mud coming toward you at the speed of a car traveling a suburban street.) These mudslides gather in volume as they travel and can carry large boulders, trees, and even cars with the flow.

Depending on the location of the landslide, it may wipe out homes or threaten human life, or both. Since landslides often dump soil and debris into bodies of water, they often create another hazard—flooding.

## CAUSES AND CURES

Land development has contributed to the potential for land-slides. Deforestation of hills as well as mining, quarrying, and road construction all interrupt the natural state of the land and diminish the underlying support. In addition, many communities pay little attention to the need to build on solid ground. While cliffs above water make for beautiful living room vistas, the likeli-hood of soil erosion underneath a home should be taken into ac-count when you're doing any type of construction. Along the Pacific coast, entire homes have slipped down hills after periods of intense rainfall.

A long-term solution to preventing some landslides involves intelligent land management: Trees, grass, and various types of vegetation need to be planted on unstable surfaces to reduce the likelihood of landslides.

## IS YOUR AREA PRONE TO LANDSLIDES?

If the area where you live is prone to landslides, you'll likely know it. Neighbors will talk of previous incidents, or you'll real-ize you're at the top (or the bottom) of a steep slope, or you'll have a drainage channel nearby. These all signify the possibility of a landslide. You can also check hillsides around your home for signs of land movement, such as small landslides or debris flows or progressively tilting trees.

If your area is vulnerable:

- Contact a private consulting company that specializes in earth movement (the company specialty might be geo-technical engineering, civil engineering, or structural en-gineering) for opinions and advice on corrective measures to take. If you aren't certain whom to contact, speak to someone in your town or county building or land use department.

- Some communities report success with trenches that catch and halt smaller landslides.
- Barriers can sometimes help divert mudflows or landslides. If you attempt to protect your own home, be sure not to divert the earth so that it flows toward the property of someone else. If damage occurs to the other person's land, you could be liable.
- Install flexible pipe fittings to avoid gas or water leaks in the event of a landslide.
- Talk to your insurance agent. Land and debris flows may be covered by flood insurance available through the National Flood Insurance Program.

## WHAT TO DO DURING A BAD STORM

- Stay alert and awake during periods of intense rainfall. Even short periods can be dangerous. Many debris-flow fatalities occur when people are sleeping.
- Evacuate if you are concerned about your area. If you decide to leave and feel you have time, notify emergency personnel (police or fire personnel), and check in with your neighbors to give them the opportunity to leave as well.

## IF YOU ARE OUTDOORS IN A LANDSLIDE-PRONE AREA

- Be particularly careful when driving. Embankments along roadsides are especially vulnerable. Watch the road for collapsed pavement, mud, fallen rocks, and other indications of debris.
- If you're near a stream or channel, be alert for any increase or decrease in water flow and for a change from clear to muddy water, which may indicate landslide activity upstream.
- If you're hiking:

- ◆ Try not to set off a landslide. Walk on high land, staying away from gullies and channels. Hikers should take slightly different paths across landslide-prone terrain. As with avalanches, you don't want to disturb the delicate nature of the soil placement in the area.
- ◆ Listen for unusual noises such as cracking trees or rocks knocking together.
- ◆ Climb to higher ground as soon as you think that the land is giving way.
- ◆ If escape is impossible, roll into a ball to try to protect your face and abdomen. Use your hands to cover the back of your neck.

## YOUR HOME AFTER A LANDSLIDE

Don't return to your home until emergency personnel have given clearance to the area. If you arrive and discover that your home seems undisturbed, you should still take the situation seriously:

- ● Have the foundation of the house checked by a contractor, and talk to a geotechnical expert to discuss additional ways to reduce landslide risk.
- ● Replant damaged ground as soon as possible; erosion caused by loss of ground cover can lead to flash flooding.

## TWO TOP TIPS TO TEACH CHILDREN ABOUT LANDSLIDES

1. If you live in a landslide-prone area, or if you take your children hiking, teach them to listen carefully for the rumble of a landslide. Then show them how to get to higher ground.
2. Teach children not to play in dry streambeds during a time

when landslides are occurring. In a landslide, a dry creek bed becomes nature's highway.

## HOT BUTTON

- If your home is vulnerable to landslides, talk to an engineer about what provisions you can make to lessen your risk. Special safety measures may earn you savings on your insurance premium.
- If you're caught in a landslide while hiking, try to get to higher ground. If escape is impossible, roll into a ball to try to protect your face and abdomen. Use your hands to cover the back of your neck.

# Lightning and Severe Thunderstorms

While moviegoers flock to action films like *Twister* and *Volcano*, Hollywood has yet to make a thriller about lightning and thunder. Maybe one day they should. Thunderstorms are more prevalent than other weather-related disasters, just as dramatic, and quite dangerous.

Thunderstorms may occur singly, in clusters, or in lines, and they last an average of 20 to 30 minutes. Wind gusts accompanying thunderstorms can sometimes reach 100–150 miles per hour, enough to flip cars, vans, and semi-trucks. Tornadoes develop from severe thunderstorms along and ahead of cold fronts, and heavy rain can lead to flash floods. The National Weather Service classifies a thunderstorm severe if it produces hail at least three-fourths of an inch in diameter, has winds of at least 58 miles per hour, or produces a tornado. However, even lesser storms can be quite dangerous.

Every thunderstorm produces lightning. In the United States, 75–100 people are killed each year by lightning—more than hurricanes and tornadoes combined—and many more are injured.

Those who do survive often report a variety of long-term debilitating symptoms, including memory loss, attention deficits, sleep disorders, numbness, dizziness, stiffness in joints, irritability, fatigue, weakness, muscle spasms, depression, and an inability to sit for long.

No state is exempt from thunderstorms and lightning, and central Florida is known as the Lightning Capital of the World. Here, severe storms occur daily during the summer. They generally pass quite quickly, but they can catch people by surprise.

## GENERAL SAFETY

In any major storm, a certain amount of damage occurs needlessly when property isn't well maintained:

- Keep trees properly trimmed. This is the single biggest mistake people make when it comes to storm preparation. Weathering a storm can be difficult in any case, but dead or dangling branches can be brought down by winds and rain, causing even more damage than necessary.
- Keep your property clear of debris. If storms are in the forecast and you're having any construction work done, ask that the contractor tarp and tie down items that could blow around in strong winds.
- If you live in a storm-prone area, have shutters installed on each window. They can be closed and latched before any major storm arrives.
- Install lightning rods where appropriate. These will carry the electrical charge safely to the ground, greatly reducing the chance of a lightning-induced fire.
- If you farm, insure crops against financial loss from storm damage through the Federal Crop Insurance Corporation of the USDA. Each year severe storms cause millions of dollars worth of crop damage, and these losses are not covered

through usual insurance policies. Hail in particular has been known to wipe out entire fields.

## BEING YOUR OWN WEATHER FORECASTER

In many parts of the country, thunderstorms move in quite quickly, and for that reason, it's important to keep one eye on the sky if you're outdoors on a day when the weather is unsettled.

- Pay attention to weather clues that may warn of danger. Look for darkening skies, flashes of light, or increasing wind, as these are signs of an approaching thunderstorm.
- Always keep an ear out for thunder, especially if you are in a vulnerable place such as a swimming pool or golf course.
- Postpone outdoor activities if a thunderstorm is moving into your area.
- Coaches of outdoor sports teams should have NOAA Weather Radios for practices and games. Team members should be sent off the field to shelter at the first sign of a thunderstorm.
- If you're outside when a storm is approaching, go inside a sturdy building or car (not a convertible). A hardtop vehicle will offer some protection.

## WHAT YOU NEED TO KNOW ABOUT LIGHTNING

According to Rocky Lopes, Disaster Services representative for the American Red Cross, most deaths from lightning can be prevented.

Lightning is nearby when the thunderclap is heard very quickly after the flash of light. If you can even hear the rumble of thunder, you are in danger of being struck by lightning. Precautions should be taken immediately. Lightning often strikes outside of heavy rain and may make contact as far as ten miles away from any rainfall, so it's important to get out of pools, begin to clear amusement park rides, and start walking out of open clearings such as golf courses or fields. What people call "heat lightning" is actually lightning from a thunderstorm too far away for the thunder to be heard but not too far away for the lightning to do damage nearby.

What's more, lightning doesn't necessarily strike the tallest object in the area; it strikes the best conductor on the ground, which is sometimes a human being. That's what makes golf courses so dangerous during a storm. In London's Hyde Park two women were killed when lightning traveled through the metal underwire in their bras.

- When there is lightning, your first priority is to seek shelter.
- Golfers need to go toward the clubhouse as quickly as possible.
- If you are boating or swimming, head for land immediately and get indoors if possible, even if the storm seems very far away. Stay away from rivers, lakes, and other bodies of water, and get off the beach. Water is an excellent conductor of electricity, and even the saturated sand conducts electricity very well. Each year people are killed by nearby lightning strikes while in the water or on the beach.

## IF YOU CAN'T GET INDOORS WHEN THERE IS LIGHTNING

- Don't take shelter under a tree or other tall object. People sometimes get shocked when the tree is hit and the electrical charge travels through the tree's root system.
- Stay away from all tall objects, including trees, towers, fences, and telephone or power lines, all of which are more likely to be struck by lightning.
- Drop anything metal that you're holding (umbrellas, base-

ball bats, fishing rods, golf clubs, camping equipment, bicycles), and come back for it later.

- If you are in the woods, find an area protected by a low clump of trees or go to a low-lying open place. Watch for flooding.
- Learn the "crouch" position. Because a lightning current often enters a victim through the ground rather than by a direct strike, the goal of the crouch is not only to become small, but also to minimize contact with the ground: *Crouch with only the balls of the feet touching the ground. Bring your head down toward your knees. Try to use your hands to cover your ears to minimize hearing damage from the thunder.*

  Some think that lying flat is the best way to avoid lightning, but don't do it. This position actually exposes more of your body to any current traveling through the ground.

- If you're with other people, split up and try to put 15 feet between each of you. If lightning hits one person, it may spread to others in a "side splash" effect.

  While it is counterintuitive to separate from children during violent weather, it's the right thing to do. You are a bigger target than they are, and if you are hit—or absorb the shock from the ground—while holding onto them, the charge will go directly into their smaller bodies. If you've practiced the "crouch" position with them in the past, just remind them of what they need to do.

## IF SOMEONE IS STRUCK BY LIGHTNING

- Get medical help as quickly as possible.
- Start first aid procedures. Begin rescue breathing if the person isn't breathing. If the person's heart has stopped, find someone to give CPR.
- If the person has a pulse and is breathing, look for other

injuries. Victims carry no electrical charge and can be handled safely:

- Check for burns in two locations. The injured person who has received an electrical shock may be burned both where the electricity entered and where it left the body.
- Being struck by lightning can also cause nervous system damage, broken bones, and loss of hearing or eyesight.

## WHAT TO DO WHEN A WARNING IS ISSUED FOR THE AREA

If a severe thunderstorm warning (warnings mean imminent developments) is issued for your area, take cover the way you would if a tornado were approaching.

- Draw blinds and shades. If a window breaks from objects blown by the wind, shades will help prevent glass from shattering.
- Select an interior room in your home where you can wait out the storm. By staying out of rooms with windows, you reduce your risk of being hurt by glass that may be broken by wind or hail.
- Avoid using the telephone or appliances during a thunderstorm. Lightning may strike exterior electric and phone lines, inducing shocks to inside equipment, including televisions and hardwired telephones. This can make these appliances dangerous during a thunderstorm. Using a wireless phone would not present any danger.
- Stay away from running water inside the house; avoid washing your hands or taking a bath or shower. Electrical currents from lightning have been known to come inside through the plumbing. Once again, modern improvements lessen the danger. If your home has PVC piping instead of

copper, lightning is less likely to enter the home through the plumbing.

- Turn off all air-conditioning units during the storm. Power surges from lightning can overload the compressor, resulting in costly repairs.

## HAIL

I grew up in Colorado, where my father ran an insurance agency. When it hailed, he never took the phone from his ear as clients, friends, and neighbors called in to report holes in their roofs, pockmarks and major damage to their automobiles, shattered windows, and ruined crops. In some parts of the country, damage from hail can be immense.

Hail can be smaller than a pea or as large as a softball, and because it comes suddenly in the midst of a thunderstorm, it can wreak havoc, destroying property and farm crops as well as injuring animals and people, from flying glass and debris.

If it begins to hail, try to get animals into shelter, and take cover yourself.

## DRIVING DURING A HEAVY RAIN

- Be sure your headlights are on, using a low beam. While the lights may not help you see the road much better, they will help other drivers see your car.
- Be aware of "hydroplaning," a dangerous situation in which the water keeps the car from making contact with the road. It's much like driving on ice. In Florida they actually have a special term, "Florida Ice," for a type of hydroplaning that occurs there. Oil and other fluids that have dripped from cars and baked into the road can come to the surface during a rainstorm and make the roads very slippery and dangerous.

- Avoid flooded roadways, being particularly careful at bridges, highway dips, and low areas. Most flood fatalities are caused by people attempting to drive through water or people playing in high water. You often can't accurately judge the water's depth. Rapidly rising water may stall the engine, engulf the vehicle and its occupants, and sweep them away. As little as two feet of water will carry away most cars.
- If you're uncomfortable driving, pull completely off the road into a parking lot or a rest area. Pulling onto the shoulder leaves you vulnerable—you could still be rear-ended by a driver who, also struggling with visibility, doesn't realize you pulled off. When you select a stopping place, try to choose an area away from trees or other tall objects that can fall onto the vehicle. Stay in the car and turn on the flashers until the storm subsides.
- Within the car, play it safe and avoid contact with metal while you wait out the storm. Lightning that strikes nearby can travel through wet ground to your car. Rubber tires provide no protection from lightning, but by avoiding contact with potential conductors (metal), you reduce your chance of being shocked. Although you may be injured if lightning strikes your car, you are better off inside than out.
- If you decide to proceed and the area is unfamiliar to you, look for a car with a local license plate. That driver may have a better sense of the road and would be a good one to follow.
- As the storm seems to be subsiding, listen to the car radio to make sure it's over and to find out about blocked roadways.
- Report downed power lines immediately.

## THREE TOP TIPS TO TEACH CHILDREN ABOUT LIGHTNING AND THUNDERSTORMS

1. Teach children they must be their own "lifeguards." If they hear thunder or see lightning when they are in the pool, they must get out immediately. It doesn't matter if the storm seems to be far away. They have to get out even if the real lifeguard hasn't blown the whistle yet—tell them it's that important.
2. Children should be taught to take cover whenever they are outside and there's thunder or a hailstorm.
3. Teach them the "crouch" position. If they can't take cover and there's lightning, they should crouch with only the balls of their feet touching the ground. Hands go on knees and the head should be kept as low as possible.

## HOT BUTTON

- If the weather seems unsettled, keep an eye out for a thunderstorm. You are your own best weather predictor. If you see that a storm is coming, head for cover.
- Practice the "crouch" position with your children.
- Wait out a severe thunderstorm in an interior room of your home, and stay away from appliances, hard-wired phones, and running water.
- When driving, be careful of hydroplaning, and don't drive on any roadway you can't see.
- If you have to pull off the road, try to find a rest area. If you have to park on the shoulder, you're vulnerable to being hit from behind.

# The Ozone Layer and the Sun

When the weather forecaster gives an Ozone Alert during the summer months, all those who have difficulty breathing know to pay attention. They realize that air quality will be poor, and they'll need to remain inside in air-conditioning as much as possible.

Unfortunately, most Americans have chosen to ignore the ever-present "Ozone Alert" concerning the dangers of the sun's rays to their skin.

## ABOUT THE OZONE SITUATION
## AND HOW IT AFFECTS US ALL

The ozone is a thin layer of gas in the stratosphere between 10 and 30 miles above the earth's surface. It makes life possible by filtering out dangerous radiation, especially ultraviolet rays, from the sun. We are dependent on it for our good health, yet many products created by man are gradually destroying this protective covering. Scientific readings reflect that an ever-increasing "hole" is occurring in the ozone, and one result is going to be an increase in the incidence of skin cancer.

Skin cancer is the most preventable of all cancers. The most serious form, malignant melanoma, claims approximately 9200 lives each year, according to the Centers for Disease Control and Prevention, and a full million more Americans per year develop some type of skin cancer. A minimum of 90 percent of those are linked to sun exposure.

While sunscreen can protect our skin, experts are convinced that it's also part of the problem. Because people feel they are protected by sunscreen, they are less cautious about prolonged exposure to the sun and less worried, too, about midday exposure.

Because melanoma numbers have continued to rise despite an increase in the use of sunscreens, experts are beginning to think that excessive sun exposure with or without sunburn (which, of course, is lessened by sunscreen) is a contributing factor to melanoma. So despite the addition of sunscreen to our arsenal of tools, it's still important to respect the damage the sun can do. Doctors want us to remember the "old-fashioned" ways of protecting our skin: covering up, wearing hats, and very simply, not staying outside for prolonged periods of time.

In the early 1990s Mt. Sinai Medical Center in New York City ran an ad that said it all: "At 5:25 this morning the leading cause of cancer appeared." Below those words was a picture of the sun.

## WHAT ABOUT THAT "HEALTHY TAN"?

The term "healthy tan" is an oxymoron. Skin that is browned or red from the sun is actually damaged skin. In an effort to gain protection from further damage, the skin cells produce a pigment called "melanin," which darkens the skin. By the time a tan develops, permanent damage has already been done and may someday show up in the form of wrinkles, blotches, sagging tissue, and even skin cancer.

Healthy skin is the color that each person's skin is naturally. As parents, one of the greatest favors we can do for our children is to work on reteaching what a "healthy" look is. The Australian government has been trying to do just this with its citizens. With the highest incidence of skin cancer in the world, Australia has run successful "sun-danger awareness" campaigns and encouraged their media to use untanned models (often wearing hats) for swimsuit models.

## WHAT ARE THOSE DIFFERENT RAYS ALL ABOUT?

Quite simply, there are two types of rays from the sun. *Ultraviolet A (UVA)* is the radiation responsible for tanning (and the type used by tanning salons for golden-bronze tans). It is the one that most directly causes aging of the skin. *Ultraviolet B (UVB)* rays are more intense than UVA. UVB causes rapid tanning as well as sunburns that are frequently associated with skin cancer. UVB exposure is strongest in spring and summer with two-thirds of the photo-damaging effects of UVB appearing between 10:00 A.M. and 4:00 P.M.

## WHAT DO THE SUNSCREEN TERMS MEAN?

Because of all the confusion over terms associated with sunscreens, the Food and Drug Administration has issued new regulations for labeling, testing, and manufacturing sun protection products. The rules do away with terms like "sunblock," "waterproof" and "all-day protection."

- **SPF (sun protection factor):** A study conducted by Britain's Health Education Authority found that only one in five people understand SPF fully. Here's how it works: If you have skin that would begin to burn after 10 minutes in the sun and are wearing sunscreen with a sun protection factor of 15, then you can stay in the sun for 150 minutes or two and a half hours without burning. To lessen the confusion, a new rating system has been developed that should be more understandable to the public: Now sunscreens will be ranked as offering "minimum," "moderate," or "high" protection. High includes any product with an SPF factor of 30 or greater; moderate is 12–29 and minimum is 2–11. Someone wearing a sunscreen of SPF 15 would take 15 times longer to burn than someone not wearing sunscreen.
- **Chemical screen versus physical:** There are two kinds of sunscreen. Chemical sunscreens penetrate the skin and absorb sunlight and are invisible on the skin. Physical sunscreens, made of titanium dioxide or zinc oxide, rest on top of the skin to create a light-reflecting shield. These may appear slightly white on the skin.

- ***Water resistant versus waterproof:*** Most sunscreens will withstand mild to moderate perspiration or swimming, but nothing is really waterproof. Under the new regulations, sunscreens will either be "water resistant" or "very water resistant."

## WHAT YOU ALREADY KNOW

- Those with light skin and eyes, or a history of severe blistering sunburns as a child, are the most at risk for skin cancer.
- Eighty percent of a person's lifetime exposure to sun happens in the first 18 years. Childhood is the time when people are more likely to spend long periods swimming and playing outdoors.
- The sun is at its strongest between 10:00 A.M. and 2:00 P.M.
- You need to cover up. Wear a hat with a four-inch brim, a long-sleeve shirt, long pants, closed shoes, and socks.

## WHAT YOU MAY NOT KNOW

- Certain fabrics allow a dangerous amount of ultraviolet radiation to pass through, and fabrics lose about one-third of their sun protective ability when they are wet. Surprisingly, a wet light-colored T-shirt transmits almost as much light as bare skin. To get the protection you need, look for loose-fitting clothes with a tight weave, and apply sunscreen even on parts of the body covered by clothing. Some companies are marketing clothing treated with sunscreen to more completely block the sun's rays. Remember that protecting your skin is a year-round affair, so when extreme heat isn't an issue, wear dark colors because they provide better skin protection than light.
- You may not be using enough sunscreen. Recent studies have indicated that people tend to underapply sunscreen

and only get 20–50 percent of the rated sun protection factor. An average woman needs about a full ounce (two tablespoons) of sunscreen spread over her body in order to be fully protected.

- A key element of using sunscreen effectively is putting it on 20–30 minutes before exposure. Applying the lotion prior to sun exposure helps lock the chemicals into the skin so that they can work effectively. Putting on sunscreen after you've already gone out into the sun is like putting on a bulletproof vest after you've been shot.
- Reapplying sunscreen is a good idea after swimming or sweating a lot, but it does not extend the time for which you're shielded. You're only protected for the number of hours you originally calculated, based on the product's sun protection factor.
- Medication increases sun sensitivity.
- On cloudy days you still need to wear sunscreen and dark glasses. Up to 80 percent of the sun's radiation can still reach us even when it's cloudy.
- Reflective surfaces (pools, open areas of concrete) can reflect up to 85 percent of the sun's damaging rays. Sitting in the shade by the pool only partially helps.

## WHAT ELSE YOU NEED TO KNOW

- Don't use sunscreen on a baby younger than six months.
- Men with thinning hair should always wear a hat or use a sunscreen on their scalp.
- Most photodamage and skin cancer occurs on the top of the head, around the eyes, nose, lips, shoulders, neck and back of the hands. Don't forget to put sunscreen on these areas.
- Reapply sunscreen every two hours when outdoors. (But remember that it doesn't extend the amount of time for which you're protected.)

- Use protective clothing, shade, and the indoors as part of your "sun protection system."
- Wear dark glasses with UV protective lenses.
- It is recommended that you check yourself monthly for signs of cancer, and see a dermatologist annually.
- To do a self-examination, examine your body front and back in the mirror, then right and left sides, arms raised. Bend your elbows and look carefully at forearms, palms, and upper arms. Next, look at the back of the legs and feet, checking the soles of your feet and between your toes. Use a hand mirror to check the back of your neck and scalp, using a blow dryer to aid with visibility on the scalp.

In general, you're looking for anything new on your skin or anything that is changing:

- Basal cell cancer usually appears as a small bump or nodule on the neck, scalp, or hand, or as a small flat growth elsewhere on the body. It doesn't spread quickly and rarely metastasizes, but should be taken care of.
- A precancerous lesion presents itself as a raised, scaly, dry patch that doesn't heal.
- Signs of melanoma include the following ABCD's:

  **A.** Asymmetry: One half of the mole doesn't match the other.
  **B.** Border irregularity: The edges of a mole are ragged, notched, or blurred.
  **C.** Color: The pigmentation isn't the same—it appears mottled in color.
  **D.** Diameter is greater than six millimeters (about one-quarter of an inch). Any sudden or continuing increase in size should be brought to the attention of a doctor.

## VACATION ALERT

The intense sunlight experienced on the first hot days of summer and during short vacations in warm climates is particularly dangerous.

## SO WHERE'S THE GOOD NEWS?

Even if you've had a great deal of sun exposure over your lifetime, you can arrest the development of most skin cancers by reducing your sun exposure now.

## KIDS AND SUNSCREENS

Getting a child to wear sunscreen regularly (and reapply it after swimming) is an art in itself, but making it as natural as brushing teeth will help a child feel as though "something is missing" if it isn't done. Here are some suggestions:

- There is a wide range of sunscreens available on the market today, from creams and lotions to sprays and gels. A child as young as seven or eight may have an opinion on what he or she wants to wear. Let that dictate what you buy. Some years kids at camp have sported purple and blue sunscreens; other times sunscreen with sparkle in it is considered "cool." Those that show up on the skin are particularly helpful when you're putting them on because you can see where the sunscreen has been applied.
- If your child doesn't currently have a preference, experiment with several different types. Though PABA is an excellent sunscreen, it causes allergies in some children. Some sunscreens feel "greasy," others are difficult to rub in—let each family member decide. It's worth the investment.

## THE IMPORTANCE OF WEARING DARK GLASSES

Chronic sun exposure is directly related to the onset of cataracts and is responsible for a sizable proportion of the more than one million cataracts that are operated on yearly. Studies have shown that people whose eyes are exposed to the sun for hours every day are three times as likely to develop cataracts than those who protect their eyes with approved sunglasses or brimmed hats. Chronic sun exposure is also linked to malignant melanomas of the eyelids, as well as macular degeneration, a leading cause of blindness.

Select glasses that block at least 99 percent of the UVA and UVB rays. (Wraparound glasses are recommended for maximum protection.) If you're not used to wearing sunglasses regularly, pick up several inexpensive pairs and keep them in your car, in your coat pockets, or in your briefcase. That way you'll have a pair wherever you need them, including cloudy days.

## THREE TOP TIPS TO TEACH CHILDREN ABOUT THE SUN

1. Tans aren't healthy. Discourage sunbathing, and make using sunscreen part of a regular routine.
2. Encourage wearing hats.
3. Children would do well to wear UV-protected sunglasses. Because of kids' active lifestyles, this often isn't practical, but help your child shop for a pair that he or she might wear some of the time.

## HOT BUTTON

- Set a good example. Protect your skin by using sunscreen, wearing protective clothing, and staying in the shade or indoors some of the time.

- Wear dark glasses whenever you're out.
- Visit a dermatologist regularly. Skin cancer is highly curable when caught early.

# Tornadoes

Today more people than ever before survive tornadoes because our warning systems are better, our homes are constructed solidly, and medical improvements are such that if a person is hurt in a tornado, emergency rescue squads are well prepared to administer first aid until the person can be placed in the capable hands of doctors.

That's not how it was a hundred years ago: At the turn of the last century, people had no warning system other than visual spotting of a storm, and there were no safety codes specifying how establishments were to be built. If a home or business was hit, the likelihood of fire from the home heating system was high. In addition, injured people had little chance of surviving because infection and gangrene so often set in before they could recover.

One of the major differences between "then" and "now" is that scientific developments have revolutionized the way weather systems can be tracked. Today it is sometimes possible for meteorologists to keep people abreast of what is happening street by street as a twister approaches, as if they were talking about yardage gained in a football game. Experts agree that the F-5 tornado that hit Oklahoma and Kansas in May of 1999 would have exacted a much higher death toll if ordinary citizens had not been able to follow its progress on television, taking cover just before the twister "came calling" on their street. Still, keep in mind that these storms are unpredictable and can change direction in seconds. If a tornado is in your area, you need to use your own judgment and stay abreast of radio and television reports.

As remarkable as their tracking ability has become, scientists are frustrated because they still can't identify what happens at the very end of the development process. At this crucial stage it is determined whether the tornado is a weak one that will fall apart quickly or a monster storm that will wreak terrible destruction. Until that piece of the puzzle falls in place, weather forecasters won't feel confident that they can warn people adequately.

In the meantime, people have learned it's important to heed tornado warnings and do what you can to protect yourself and your family from what can be the most violent atmospheric phenomenon on the planet.

## ABOUT TORNADOES

A tornado is a violently rotating column of air extending from a thunderstorm to the ground. The strongest tornadoes have rotating winds of 250 miles per hour or more. They are capable of causing extreme destruction, including uprooting trees and well-made structures, and turning normally harmless objects into deadly missiles. Most tornadoes are just a few dozen yards wide and only briefly touch down, but highly destructive, violent tornadoes may carve out paths over a mile wide and more than 50 miles long.

Tornadoes usually develop from severe thunderstorms in warm, moist, unstable air along and ahead of cold fronts. Such thunderstorms also may generate large hail, dangerous lightning, and other damaging winds. (Tropical storms and hurricanes that hit land also generate tornadoes.)

Scientist T. Theodore Fujita created a tornado "intensity" scale with 12 rankings from F-0 to F-11, but wind speeds and intensities above F-5 have never been documented. F-0 and F-1 tornadoes are weak systems with winds of 40–112 miles an hour; an F-3 storm's winds are 158 to 206 miles an hour; F-4 and F-5 signify the strongest systems with wind speeds of more than 206 miles an hour.

Tornadoes typically last only 2–3 minutes, but the ones that do major damage probably average about 15 minutes.

While you sometimes hear reference to "Tornado Alley," there are actually several. According to The Tornado Project, the area from central Texas to Colorado, North Dakota, and Minnesota is one; another tornado-prone area extends eastward from Texas to Georgia, and still another runs from Arkansas to the Ohio River and the Great Lakes states of Ohio, Indiana, Illinois, and Michigan. Southern New England (western Massachusetts and Connecticut) also get more than their fair share of tornadoes. But no area should consider itself immune. There are occasional tornadoes in mountain areas, in Hawaii, and in California, areas where one might least expect to encounter a tornado.

About half the tornadoes that occur in the world happen in the United States, and though there are areas in which tornadoes are more common, tornadoes can and do occur at any time and in almost any place. One of the worst tornadoes in history occurred in Massachusetts, and Florida gets more small tornadoes per square mile than any other state. Though most occur in late afternoon and evening, they can pop up at any time; some of the most deadly have formed at night when no one could see them coming.

## VISUAL WARNINGS

The following weather clues may warn of imminent danger:

- a dark, often greenish sky.
- a wall cloud or funnel cloud. A visible rotating extension of the cloud base is a sign that a tornado may develop. Sometimes one or more of the clouds turns greenish (a phenomenon caused by hail), indicating that a tornado may develop.
- a cloud of debris. An approaching cloud of debris can

mark the touchdown of a tornado even if a funnel is not visible.

- roaring noise. The high winds of a tornado can cause a roar that is often compared with the sound of a rushing waterfall, jet airplane, or freight train.
- large hail, particularly if there is a "watch" or "warning" posted. Tornadoes are spawned from powerful thunderstorms, the most powerful of which produce large hail. Tornadoes frequently emerge from the hail-producing portion of the storm.
- a calm before the storm. Winds may die down and the air may become very still just before a tornado hits.

Particularly in the Great Plains, tornadoes may occur near the trailing edge of a thunderstorm and be quite visible. It is not uncommon to see clear, sunlit skies behind a tornado. They may also be embedded in rain and not be visible at all.

One of the most dangerous aspects of tornadoes is the fact that they often occur in groups. More than seven together is known as a "family." Even if one storm has passed by your neighborhood, you should be on guard for the possibility of another arising. On January 21, 1999, 38 tornadoes—the most ever to strike a state in a single day—touched down in Arkansas, killing 8 people and injuring 55.

## A WATCH VERSUS A WARNING

A "watch" means that there is a possibility that a tornado will hit your area. Locate family members, start paying attention to weather reports, and keep an eye out the window. At the first word from the weather service, or if you see anything suspicious out the window, gather family members and pets and take cover.

A "warning" is posted when a tornado has actually been spotted or is strongly indicated on radar. You should seek shelter immediately.

## WHAT TO PREPARE FOR AND WHAT TO REMEMBER

While stories of people being sucked up by the wind are frightening and true, it's most important to protect yourself from flying debris. When you take into account the harm that can come to you from being walloped by a falling branch or hit by flying glass, you quickly realize that an F-0 (the weakest rank of tornado) holds the power to be almost as dangerous as an F-5 (the strongest).

Whether you're at work, the mall, or at home when a tornado hits, there is a very specific set of actions that can save your life. If you want an easy way to remember, think "QUID."

*Think quickly*—there's no time to waste with a tornado on the ground.

*Think under*—you want to be under something if you can.

*Think in*—you want to be deep inside if at all possible.

*Think down*—once inside, go to the lowest floor possible, preferably the basement.

Remember it as *QUID.*

*Move quickly, under, in, and down.*

## HOUSE AND YARD PREP

- The safest place to wait out a storm is underground or as low to the ground as possible. If you don't have a cellar or basement, consider designating an interior hallway or a bathroom on the lowest floor as your tornado "spot." Putting as many walls between you and the outside provides additional protection. (Less than 2 percent of all tornadoes are powerful enough to completely destroy a sturdy building.) Select an area with no windows or doors, and keep the area uncluttered.
- If your locality is particularly tornado-prone, you may want

to build a "safe room" in your basement. Reinforcing some of the walls can enhance your safety.

- Some people take refuge in the bathroom because all the framing and piping lends a certain stability to the room. Because the bathtub is anchored directly into the ground, it is often one of the few things left standing. Getting into the tub with a couch cushion over you offers protection on all sides as well as an extra anchor to the foundation, but a basement is still better.

  Some people used to think that a mattress was the best thing to use for protection. However, in the May 1999 tornadoes in Oklahoma, several people were killed when they delayed getting to safety while struggling with their mattresses, and in the 1988 tornado in Andover, Kansas, three children were smothered beneath a mattress. Couch cushions offer protection without the dangers presented by mattresses.

- Consider installing permanent shutters over windows. Shutters can be closed quickly and provide the safest protection for windows.

- Strengthen garage doors to keep the wind out.

- Designate a shelf for heavy bedspreads or blankets to use for body protection. You won't have time to get these once a warning has gone out, but by having these or a couch cushion to put over you, you can protect yourself against the lighter debris that may be blowing about.

- In the yard:

  - Keep trees and shrubs trimmed. This helps make them more wind resistant and weaker branches are less likely to be blown off and cause additional damage.
  - Make a list of items to bring inside in the event of a storm.
  - Remove debris and loose items in your yard if there is time. Firewood and outdoor furniture can become missiles.

- Learn about your community's warning systems and explain them to your children. Some towns use sirens, or you may be dependent on an NOAA Weather Radio with a tone-alert feature to keep you aware of warnings and watches while you are indoors.
- Check with your workplace and your children's schools to learn tornado emergency plans. Every building has different safe places, and it's important to know how to get to them in an emergency.
- All family members should know the name of your county so everyone will understand the nature of the announcements.
- Conduct tornado drills. Practice going to your safe place so that the reaction is automatic. With children, carefully distinguish between a fire meeting place and a tornado safe place—two totally different places.

## TAKE COVER!

- Once a tornado warning has been issued, you will only have a few moments to get to safety. Gather family members and call in pets if you can. Take a cell phone if you have one.
- Go to the basement or storm cellar, or on the lowest floor of the building you are in, and try to get into an interior room or a closet. Stay away from windows and doors.
- Get under something protective—a piece of furniture such as a table or desk is ideal, but a pillow, cushion, or hardcover book is better than nothing. Try to protect your neck and head from flying or falling objects, with your arms and hands if necessary.
- It used to be thought that opening a window in the home would somehow protect against the roof blowing off. This is not only untrue, but also dangerous. The time spent opening a window is time wasted in getting yourself and family members to a safe spot. It doesn't work, so don't bother.

Rocky Lopes of the American Red Cross notes: "If a tornado wants your windows open, it will do so by itself without your help."

## IF YOU ARE IN A HIGH-RISE BUILDING

- Select a place in a hallway in the center of the building as your safe place. You may not have time to get down to a lower floor, and center hallways are often structurally reinforced.

## IF YOU'RE IN A PUBLIC BUILDING
## (SCHOOL, THEATER, STADIUM, MALL)

Your risk increases in a public building. Wide-span roofs are frequently damaged or destroyed in tornado-force winds. The supports over theaters and stadiums are often wide, and there's a lot of debris to blow around if the building is disturbed.

- If storms are in the area, skip the theater for the evening and delay your trip to the mall. Schools try to dismiss in advance to get children home before a storm.
- If, however, you're caught in a tornado, react quickly by looking for any type of cellar or basement area (QUID—quick, under, in, down). If one isn't available, choose an interior wall (under a staircase, in a closet) in which to ride out the storm. Again, crouch or lie flat under anything you can find, and cover your head with your arms and hands.
- Get out of gyms, auditoriums, and other free-span rooms. Try to get to a smaller interior room or hall, preferably on a lower floor.

## IF YOU'RE IN A CAR, A BUS, OR A TRUCK

No matter how heavy the vehicle, it's no match for many tornadoes. *Don't try to outdrive the storm.* (Storm chasers who specifically follow storms are equipped with all the latest warning devices and know which way the storm is moving and how fast—luxuries denied to you in your car.) It is not unusual for a tornado to pick up a car or truck and flip it as the storm goes by. During the storm that hit Oklahoma in May of 1999, a witness noted that dozens of cars and trucks weighing several tons each were "tossed like toys" everywhere.

- Get out of your car immediately, and remember: QUID. If there is a building nearby that is likely to be open, go inside and look for a way to go to a cellar or basement. If not, find an interior location away from windows or glass partitions, and get under something if possible. If not, then cover your head with your arms and hands and crouch or lie down.
- If you're on a highway with no nearby structures, stop your car and look for a ditch to lie in (think down, think under). Avoid being near trees as the high winds may uproot them or break off large branches. Lightning is also common during tornadoes, another reason to avoid trees.
- *Don't seek cover under highway underpasses.* A misconception has led people to believe that climbing up underneath an underpass is a safe strategy. Unfortunately, countless lives have been lost because of this misunderstanding. When a tornado is in the area, *always think down*.

## IF YOU LIVE IN A MOBILE HOME

Mobile homes are so often hit by tornadoes that some people have described trailer parks as "attracting tornadoes." Mobile homes can be flipped over easily even in rather weak tornadoes. A light trailer may be flipped by a 60 mph gust; an anchored one may sustain winds up to about 110 miles per hour. Had there been no trailer parks in their paths, some tornadoes might have been viewed as "high winds," but they're correctly identified as tornadoes as they cavalierly flip the mobile homes in their pathways.

- Because you are more at risk if you live in a mobile home, the best investment you can make is to rent space for your trailer in a mobile home park with an emergency shelter. Some parks have steel reinforced concrete laundry rooms that also offer protection.
- At the first sign of a tornado, you, your family members, and your pets (if you can get them quickly) should all go directly to the shelter.

## THE AFTERMATH

- Listen to the radio, TV, or NOAA Weather Radio for further information and instructions. You may find that all is well outside, or that roads are blocked and the area around you is devastated.
- Use the telephone for emergency calls only.
- Don't return to a damaged area until emergency personnel have given you permission to do so.
- Wear sturdy shoes and walk carefully. Injuries from stepping on shards of glass and broken objects are common following a disaster.
- Watch out for fallen power lines or broken gas lines, and report them immediately.
- Stay away from disaster areas. Your presence may hamper rescue and emergency operations.
- Use battery-powered lanterns or flashlights (not candles) when examining your home or office building.
- Look for fire dangers (gas lines, damaged electrical systems, spilled flammables). Fire is the most frequent hazard following other disasters. If you note sparks, frayed wires, or

burning insulation, shut off the electricity at the main box. If there's water in the basement, call an electrician for advice. Electrical equipment should be checked and dried before returning it to service.

- Check for gas leaks. If you smell gas or hear a blowing or hissing noise, open a window and quickly leave the building. If you can, turn off the gas at the main valve and go to a neighbor's to call the gas company.
- Take pictures of the damage to the building and its contents for insurance claims.

## THREE TOP TIPS TO TEACH CHILDREN ABOUT TORNADOES

1. Be sure children understand that a tornado "safe place" is in a cellar or an interior room. A fire "safe place" will be outside the home. Practice with them to be sure they understand.
2. Teach them to pay attention to visual cues for tornadoes. Take cover immediately if there is a warning, or if you have a sighting. Think QUID: quickly, under, in, and down.
3. If you're outside, get inside. If you can't, lie flat until the funnel passes.

## HOT BUTTON

- Usually your greatest danger in a tornado is from blowing debris. Do what you can to get underneath something or at least protect your head.
- If you're in a public building and can't get to a basement, look for an interior spot with walls.
- Get to the edge (under stairs? in a closet?) of any building with a wide-span roof.
- If you're in your car, never try to outrun a twister. You have

no way to determine which direction it will take, and you certainly can't outdrive it.

- Don't make the mistake others have made of climbing up under highway underpasses. You're safest at ground level or below.

# Tsunamis

Since 1946 six tsunamis have killed more than 350 people and damaged a half billion dollars' worth of property in Hawaii, Alaska, and on the West Coast. If you live in one of these areas, you may experience a tsunami at some point.

Tsunamis are a series of overpowering waves that occur following an earthquake or volcanic eruption, either of which may have occurred on the other side of the world or under the sea. They are potentially dangerous, and warnings of a tsunami should be heeded immediately because of the serious risk of sudden coastal flooding. However, seriously damaging tsunamis occur infrequently. Learn about them, know what to do, but don't sleep in a wet suit waiting for the next one.

## ABOUT THE TSUNAMI

Tsunamis are ocean waves produced by earthquakes, underwater landslides, or volcanic eruptions. They most frequently come ashore as a rapidly rising, turbulent surge of water choked with debris. The net result is a sudden flood that comes from the ocean.

Tsunamis may be locally generated or they may come from a distance, and their ability to destroy varies widely. In 1957 a distant-source tsunami generated by an earthquake in the Aleutian Islands in Alaska struck Hawaii 2100 miles away. Hawaii experienced $5 million in damages. In contrast, in 1992 the Cape Mendocino, California, earthquake produced a tsunami that reached Eureka in about 20 minutes and Crescent City in 50 minutes. This tsunami had a wave height of only one foot and was not destructive.

A tsunami is often incorrectly referred to as a tidal wave, but it's actually a series of waves that can travel at speeds averaging 450 and up to 600 miles per hour in the open ocean.

Ironically, tsunamis are not felt in ships because the wave length is hundreds of miles long with an amplitude of only a few feet. However, as a tsunami approaches land and the speed reduces, the amplitude increases. While waves as high as 100 feet have been recorded, generally the waves are 10–20 feet high. They can still be very destructive.

Areas most likely to suffer from a tsunami are those that are less than 25 feet above sea level and within one mile of the shoreline.

The biggest risks associated with a tsunami are those from flooding—contamination of water, property damage, or fires from ruptured gas lines—combined with the threat of drowning because of the very suddenness of the wave. The lack of predictability as to where and when a tsunami will hit is also problematic. One community may experience no damaging waves while another one an ocean away may be devastated.

## WHAT TO DO IF YOU LIVE IN A COASTAL AREA

- Town planning is important in these areas, and communities should avoid putting critical facilities (hospitals, schools, police stations, or petroleum-storage tank farms) in coastal locations.
- If you live near the coastline, elevating your home will help to reduce damage. If that isn't practical, consult an engineer for ways to make your home more resistant to water.
- Refer to the "Floods and Flash Floods" section of this book and follow flood preparedness guidelines. Also refer to Chapter Five, "Insuring Against Disaster" to be certain you have adequate insurance coverage.
- Plan an evacuation route from your home, school, office, or

any other place where you might be. Pick a destination (a friend or relative's home?) that is 100 feet or more above sea level, or one that is at least two miles inland. If you can't get this high or far, go as high as you can. Every foot inland or upward makes a difference.
● Practice your evacuation route.


## POSSIBLE SIGNS OF A TSUNAMI

● The following events might warn you of a tsunami:

◆ an earthquake near the coast, particularly one lasting 20 seconds or more.
◆ a noticeable rise or fall of coastal water—this is nature's warning system.

If either of these situations occur, you may want to consider evacuating immediately, particularly if you have dependents with special needs (the elderly, people with disabilities).

● There are also two tsunami centers whose warnings you should heed:

◆ The West Coast/Alaska Tsunami Warning Center (WC/ATWC) is responsible for tsunami warnings for California, Oregon, Washington, British Columbia, and Alaska.
◆ The Pacific Tsunami Warning Center (PTWC) is responsible for warnings to international authorities, Hawaii, and U.S. territories within the Pacific basin. They also coordinate information being disseminated.

● There are three levels of warning:

◆ An advisory means that an earthquake has occurred in the Pacific basin, and it might generate a tsunami.

WC/ATWC and PTWC will issue hourly bulletins advising of the situation.

◆ A watch indicates a tsunami may have been generated, but there is at least two hours travel time to the area in watch status. Local officials should prepare for possible evacuation.

◆ A warning indicates that a tsunami has been generated and could cause damage, so people in the area are strongly advised to evacuate.

● Listen to the radio if you notice anything unusual, or if an advisory, a watch, or a warning is issued.

## VACATION ALERT

● If you are visiting an area at risk for tsunamis, check with the hotel, motel, or campground operators for evacuation information as well as information on how you would be warned.

## IF A WARNING IS ISSUED

● Leave low-lying coastal areas.
● Don't go to the beach to watch for a tsunami. Once you can see the wave, it's too late to escape it.
● Pay attention to emergency personnel. With a tsunami, there may not be a moment to waste.
● If time permits, secure unanchored objects around your home or business.
● Tune into NOAA Weather Radio, Coast Guard emergency frequency station, or other reliable sources for updated information. Evacuate at once if they say to do so.

## AFTER A TSUNAMI

- Continue listening for weather updates on the radio so that you'll know what's happened in the rest of the region and if you've evacuated, when it's safe to return to your community.
- If you're at home, open the windows to begin to dry things out.
- Once you're ready to venture out, wear sturdy shoes.
- Use the telephone only for emergency calls.
- As with any type of flooding, stay out of buildings until you're given permission to enter, and use caution as you go in.
- Throw away all food that may have been damaged, and drink tap water only after local health officials advise that it's safe.

## ONE TOP TIP TO TEACH CHILDREN ABOUT TSUNAMIS

A tsunami warning should be taken seriously. Once one is issued, join family members at your designated meeting spot so the family can head for higher ground immediately.

## HOT BUTTON

- Take precautions similar to those you would take to prepare for a flood.
- Plan your evacuation route, and practice it.

# Volcanic Eruptions

If you were to take the scenic boat trip that goes past the magnificent smoldering beauty of the world's most active volcano, Kilauea, in Hawaii, you would be hard-pressed to understand the violent destruction that an active volcano can trigger.

To appreciate that, one need only hear about Mount St. Helens, a volcano that erupted in our own backyard. On March 27, 1980, when earthquake tremors from a quake that had occurred earlier in the week finally caused the mountain to blow a 250-foot crater out of its top, the massive amount of ash and smoke spewed forth was only the beginning. That particular eruption lasted 5½ hours, and with all the shifting that followed, by April 8, the crater measured a mile across and 850 feet deep.

Over a period of weeks, the area was assaulted by various forms of destruction: There were additional earthquakes and a mudslide (lahar) that destroyed at least 200 homes, some of which were up to 40 miles away. Ash blew throughout the area, choking the Columbia River with sediment that stalled boats and killed fish. Air and car transportation came to a halt because of gummed-up motors and poor visibility. At one point, a 500 degree steam explosion shot into the air, killing loggers who were working nine miles from the volcano. Trees were flattened, wiping out the logging industry in the area, and wildlife by the millions died. Vegetation over 230 square miles of land was totally destroyed.

## ABOUT VOLCANOES

There are over 600 active volcanoes in the world, and the United States is third in the world, after Japan and Indonesia, for the number of active volcanoes. Here, eruptions are most likely to occur in Hawaii and Alaska. In the Cascade Range in Washington, Oregon, and California, eruptions are generally limited to only one to two per century.

Volcanoes act like vents through which molten rock escapes to the earth's surface. Unlike other mountains, which are pushed up from below, volcanoes are built from the surface accumulation of their eruptive products—layers of lava, ash flows, and ash. One way geologists predict eruptions is by studying earthquake activity beneath or near active volcanoes. If there's an earthquake below a volcano, it may mean that pressure is building up and an eruption will soon occur.

Eruptions can be relatively quiet, producing lava flows that creep across the land at two to ten miles per hour; or they can be explosive, shooting columns of gases and rock fragments tens of miles into the atmosphere and spreading ash hundreds of miles downwind.

Volcanic hazards include gases, lava, and pyroclastic flows, landslides, earthquakes, and explosive eruptions. These eruptions can endanger people and property hundreds of miles away and even affect the global climate. Volcanoes are often accompanied by other natural hazards—earthquakes, mudflows, and flash floods, rockfalls and landslides, wildfires and under special conditions, tsunamis.

## JUST IN CASE . . .

The first thing to determine, of course, is whether or not there is any chance of volcano activity in your area. If you live within 100 miles of an active volcano, then you're at risk:

- Ask about community warning systems.
- Talk to your insurance agent.
- Review your evacuation plan, and ask about the evacuation plans for your children's schools.

## EMERGENCY SUPPLIES

Add to your disaster kit and your evacuation kit the following items for emergencies:

- A pair of goggles and a safety breathing mask for each member of the household in case of ashfall. A cloth that can be dampened in a mixture of water and vinegar and tied around the nose and mouth will also work as a breathing mask.
- An old set of clothing for each family member—anything with padding is best, but long sleeves and long pants to protect the skin against ash are a must.
- Helmets. Try putting aside old or unused bike helmets for this purpose.
- Extra air filters for your home and car. If the ash blows in your direction, it will quickly clog existing filters.

## SIGNS OF VOLCANIC ACTION

If you note the following signs, you'll want to leave the area immediately:

- audible rumblings from the volcano or ground
- ash and gases appearing from the cone, the sides, or around the volcano
- a change in ground temperature may indicate that the hot magma is rising
- earth movement, whether in tremors or an earthquake
- presence of pumice dust in the air
- acid rain
- steam in clouds over the mouth of the volcano
- rotten egg smell near rivers, indicating the presence of sulphur

## EVACUATION

- Evacuate the moment you're told to.
- Have all family members put on protective clothing, including sturdy shoes. Face masks, helmets, and goggles should be used if ash is in the area; if not, have each family member (except for the younger ones) hold on to their protective gear until it's needed.
- Avoid areas downwind and river valleys downstream of the volcano. Debris and ash will be carried by wind and gravity, and you want to stay in areas where you will not be exposed to volcanic hazards.
- Be prepared for difficult travel. If your car gets bogged down in ash, you may have to leave it. Then walk to the nearest road you know of and try to get a ride.
- Beware of mudflows near stream channels. They move faster than a person can run and may pull down even a building.

## WHERE TO GO

- If possible, go to an emergency shelter; those underground are best. Remember that ash can layer an area so thickly that it can cause a building to collapse. However, in a fast-moving cloud of gas or ash rock fragments, you may have very little choice.
- If you are inside when your area is blanketed by volcanic ash, stay inside until you're notified that it's safe to come out:

  - Close all windows, doors, and dampers to keep ash from entering.
  - Bring in animals and livestock.
  - Cover and protect or bring in machinery.
  - Keep an eye on ash buildup on the roof and keep an ear

peeled for sounds of creaking. You may have to get out if collapse seems imminent.

- If outdoors, seek shelter indoors. Again, an underground emergency shelter is preferable. If you can't get to it, remain aware of other potential problems you may encounter.
- If caught in a rockfall, roll into a ball to protect your head and throat.
- If caught near a stream, be aware of mudflows, particularly if you hear a roaring sound.
- Stay away from government-declared restricted zones. Mudflows, flash floods, wildfires, and even hot ash can reach you even miles away. With Mount St. Helens, the curious found it difficult to stay away, but investigating can be extremely dangerous. One of the scientists studying Mount St. Helens was killed when an eruption caught him by surprise.
- Avoid river valleys and low-lying areas.
- Follow emergency broadcasts.

## THE AFTERMATH

- Seek out those in the area who need help.
- Keep your mouth and nose covered.
- Clear roofs of ashfall. It's heavy and can cause buildings to collapse, particularly if it gets wet in the rain.
- Avoid driving in heavy ashfall. If you're caught, turn off the engine. It will clog.
- If you have a respiratory ailment, avoid all contact with ash. Stay indoors until officials advise that it's okay to go outside again.

## ONE TOP TIP TO TEACH CHILDREN ABOUT VOLCANOES

Even if helmets and masks are uncomfortable, it's important to wear them for protection.

## HOT BUTTON

- Evacuate as soon as you're instructed to.
- Stay downwind of the blowing ash.
- As fascinating as it is, don't be tempted to cross boundaries to "have a quick look" at an active volcano.

# Winter Storms

For most people a winter storm is more of an inconvenience than a serious danger. The schools may close, the roads may be difficult to navigate, and it may be really cold when you go out to shovel the walk, but after a day or two it's back to "business as usual."

However, each winter some communities find themselves in a much more treacherous predicament with a storm that becomes incapacitating. People are trapped inside for a prolonged period of time, giving rise to "cabin fever"; snow and ice may pull down power lines, creating a dangerous environment outside and a cold, uncomfortable one inside; food supplies to an area can be reduced; people in need of health care can have difficulty getting help; and as people begin to move out and about, they may encounter bitter temperatures and ice hazards.

While few people die as a direct result of a winter storm, many die from related accidents. The leading cause of death during winter storms is from car or other transportation mishaps. Exhaustion and heart attacks caused by overexertion are the two other most likely causes of winter storm-related deaths.

Like every other type of weather condition, preparation is key. You and your family can enjoy more of the beauty and less of the burden of snowy weather by taking proper precautions.

## PREPARING FOR WINTER

- In warmer weather, investigate whether there are any areas of your home where you need additional insulation.
- If you've had a problem with freezing pipes, consult your plumber before the cold weather sets in. There may be a way to add insulation to some pipes. If the pipes that are freezing are part of the heating system, your plumber may even recommend adding antifreeze to the system.
- Install storm windows.
- If you live in a rural area, consider installing snow fences to reduce drifting in roads and pathways.
- Make certain that any supplementary heating sources you plan to use are approved and safe. Portable space heaters should be tip-proof, and the heating element should be designed so that it isn't exposed. An exposed heating element might burn a person who passes by the heater or ignite a piece of clothing that comes up against it.
- House fires are more common in the winter due to a lack of correct safety precautions—unattended fires, too quick disposal of hot ash, or improperly placed space heaters are just some examples. Check your smoke alarms and add them to areas where you feel they are needed. Fire during winter storms is particularly dangerous because the water may freeze, hampering firefighters.
- Check out your snow removal equipment before the winter storm season. A gas-powered blower should not be stored with gasoline in it, and once it has gas in it again, the motor needs to be started every few weeks so that the engine doesn't gum up.

- Talk to your insurance agent about coverage. If a winter thaw could be severe enough to cause flooding, you may want to purchase coverage through the NFIP. (See Chapter Five, "Insuring Against Disaster.")

## EXTRA WINTER SUPPLIES

Before the weather turns cold, be sure you have the following:

- Warm coat, gloves or mittens, hat, and water-resistant boots for all family members
- Extra blankets and warm clothing.
- A well-stocked pantry with soups, canned fruits, and other types of food the family likes. If you can't get out for a few days, you will be glad to have extras on hand.
- Nonclumping kitty litter, which can provide temporary traction on ice and snow.

## ONCE THE SNOW STARTS

- Throughout the winter season, make it a general rule not to drive with less than a half tank of gas. A well-filled tank keeps the fuel line from freezing, and you'll be certain to have gas in an emergency.
- Before a winter storm, contact the Red Cross or your local EMA office regarding designated public shelters in case you lose power or heat.
- If you live in a rural area and have animals:

  - move animals to sheltered areas
  - have extra feed on hand
  - have a water supply available (most animal deaths in winter storms are caused by dehydration)

- If pipes are in danger of freezing, let the faucets drip a little to keep the water moving.
- If pipes freeze, call a plumber. Open all faucets, and if possible, pour hot water over the pipes. You might also attempt to warm the pipes using a handheld hair dryer, but keep in mind that this small household appliance may quickly overheat.


## KEEPING YOU AND YOUR FAMILY SAFE

- Stay inside during a snowstorm, and follow the news so that you'll be aware of the severity of the storm. Long periods of exposure to severe cold increases the risk of frostbite or hypothermia, and it's easy to become disoriented in blowing snow.
- If your dog must go out during a storm, use a leash and keep him or her with you right by the house. In upstate New York a young boy went out to search the area when the family dog didn't come back inside during a snowstorm. The dog eventually came back, but the boy didn't. By the time rescuers found him, he had died of hypothermia.
- Eat regularly to have energy for producing heat:

  - ◆ Replenish the body with water and broth and juices to keep from dehydrating.
  - ◆ Avoid alcohol and caffeine. Caffeine accelerates the symptoms of hypothermia. Alcohol hastens the effect of the cold and slows circulation, making you less aware of the effect of freezing temperatures.

- Conserve fuel. Great demand may be placed on electricity, gas, and other fuel distribution systems. If your heat is dependent on your receiving regular oil deliveries, it's extremely important to preserve what you have. The oil companies may have difficulty arriving on schedule. Set the thermometer at 65 during the day and 55 at night. Close unused rooms, and cover windows at night.

## IF YOU MUST GO OUT

- Warm your body by stretching before you go out. If you're shoveling snow, this will reduce the risk of muscle injury.
- Dress in layers and wear a hat and mittens. Layered clothing provides better insulation than a single warm piece of clothing, and since most body heat is lost through the head, be sure to wear a hat. Keep hands and feet warm, too. Mittens are warmer than gloves, and a scarf protects the lungs from extremely cold air.
- Keep dry. If you get wet while out, change frequently. Wet clothing transmits heat rapidly away from the body.
- Take frequent breaks to warm up, and avoid overexertion from shoveling heavy snow, pushing a car, or walking in deep snow. The strain from the cold and the hard labor may cause a heart attack. Too much sweating can lead to chills and hypothermia.
- Walk carefully on snowy, icy sidewalks. Slips and falls occur frequently in winter weather and can cause a disabling injury.
- If you're leaving your home, use public transportation if possible. About 70 percent of winter deaths related to ice and snow occur in automobiles.
- Understand the hazards of windchill, a calculation of how cold it feels when the effects of wind speed and temperature are combined. As the wind increases, heat is carried away from a person's body at an accelerated rate, driving down body temperature. Even with a not-so-cold temperature on the thermometer, the windchill factor can create a situation that's cold enough to cause hypothermia.

# IF YOU'RE WITHOUT HEAT FOR
# AN EXTENDED PERIOD

If bad weather has cut the power to your home or apartment for more than a day or so, you might be concerned about how long you will be able to tolerate the dropping inside temperatures.

Your home or apartment house will hold some heat, but the amount retained will depend on how well the building is insulated and for how long you're without a furnace. Access to a fireplace or a wood-burning stove, of course, makes this condition far more tolerable. If there is no heating source at all, a normally healthy person can tolerate a cold home by taking a few precautions:

- In an apartment or home without a fireplace, select one room for all family members. Choose an interior room (or one without many windows) that is small enough to hold some of the body heat generated, but large enough for the family to be comfortable—a bedroom or a dining room is a good choice.
- Bring in extra blankets. Use some to seal off under-door breezes; use the remainder to keep people warm.
- Everyone should dress in layered clothing and hats. The air space between the clothing layers acts as insulation, and hats help maintain the large proportion of body heat that people otherwise lose through their heads.
- Special attention should be paid to keeping feet and hands warm as the extremities are more prone to frostbite. Wear warm shoes and gloves, and move around often, stamping feet and clapping hands to keep up body circulation. Sandwiching your fingers in the pit of your arms (inside your coat) will also help keep them warm.
- Take turns sleeping in short shifts. At least one person should be awake at all times just to make sure everyone is okay.

• When should you leave for a shelter or another location? This is a decision you must make based on your particular circumstances. If the shelter or a heated home is relatively close and the outdoor conditions are cold, but the snow is gone, then you might consider it. However, if the roads are bad, you increase the odds of getting injured in a crash or getting stuck on the road. In general, there is merit to staying put. The problems that await you in a frozen, snow-covered world may be worse than waiting out the storm in a very chilly home or apartment.

If someone has a health condition, is elderly or very young, arrangements should be made before a storm strikes to go somewhere else for shelter. In some communities, local emergency managers or local public health authorities collect the names and phone numbers of people at particular risk. In situations where the power may be out for an extended period, an attempt is made to provide transportation to a warm shelter for those people. Check with your municipal government or contact the Senior Center in your area for more information.

## HYPOTHERMIA AND FROSTBITE

If you start to shiver a lot or get very tired, or if your nose, fingers, toes, or earlobes start to feel numb or turn very pale, come inside right away. These are signs of hypothermia and frostbite. You will need immediate attention.

Hypothermia is brought on when body temperature drops to less than 95°F. Symptoms include uncontrollable shivering, slow speech, memory lapses, frequent stumbling, drowsiness, and exhaustion. Hypothermia is not always fatal but for those who survive, there is likely to be lasting kidney, liver, and pancreas damage.

Frostbite is a severe reaction to cold exposure that can cause permanent harm. A loss of feeling and a white or pale appearance in fingers, toes, nose or earlobes are symptoms of frostbite.

If frostbite or hypothermia is suspected, begin warming the person slowly and seek immediate medical assistance. Warm the person's trunk first. Using your own body heat will help. Arms and legs should be warmed last because stimulation of the limbs can drive cold blood toward the heart and lead to heart failure. Put the person in dry clothing and wrap their entire body in a blanket. Never give them alcohol or caffeine. Caffeine can cause the heart to beat faster and hasten the effect the cold has on the body. Alcohol, a depressant, can slow the heart and also hasten the ill effects of the cold.

Elderly people account for the largest percentage of hypothermia victims. Many older Americans literally "freeze to death" in their homes after being exposed to dangerously cold temperatures, or are asphyxiated because of improper use of fuels such as charcoal briquettes, which produce carbon monoxide.

## PREPARING YOUR CAR FOR WINTER

When it comes to the mechanics of car operation, winter is the most difficult time of year. Get your car tuned up in September or early October so that you're prepared for the first significant snowfall:

- Get your battery, lights, ignition, and brake system checked.
- Add antifreeze to your heating and cooling systems, as well as the washer solvent for the windshield wipers.
- Check to make certain the heater and defroster are working properly. If you store antifreeze at home, do so carefully— it's highly poisonous, and because it's sweet, kids and pets are attracted to it.
- Consider what to do about your tires. All-weather radials are adequate for most winter conditions. However, some ju-

risdictions require that vehicles be equipped with chains or snow tires with studs.

- During cold weather, carry a book of matches in your coat pocket or purse. If your car lock freezes, use the match to warm the key. Insert the key in the lock, and then wait for a moment while the heated key melts the ice. (If you turn the key too soon, you might bend it.)

### Items to Add to the Trunk of Each Car for the Winter:

- Check that your flashlight is still in the car, and add extra batteries
- Small snow shovel
- Small bag of sand, salt, or kitty litter
- Ice scraper and brush
- Tow chain
- Traction mats
- Flatboard to create a firm base for the jack stand
- Candle and waterproof matches (a lit candle in a three-pound coffee can will produce a fair degree of heat)

### The Following Items Should Be Added If a Storm Is in Progress or Predicted and You Have to Travel Anyway:

- A well-charged cell phone.
- Quick-energy foods such as chocolate or dried fruits will help produce body heat.
- One to two bottles of drinking water.
- Thermal blankets and extra clothing, gloves, hats, and boots. Any essential prescription medicine should be added to the first aid kit in case you are stranded for a period of time.
- Seasoned drivers also pack a thermos of hot soup before each trip.

## VENTURING OUT?

When the weather is poor, experts advise that you should always ask yourself, "Is this trip really necessary?" If you must go, plan to remain on well-traveled roads where cars pass frequently. Advise family members and friends of your route, destination, and any changes in your travel plans. Don't rush.

## DRIVING DURING A STORM

- Don't warm up a car in a closed garage.
- If your car has been parked outside, clean snow and ice off completely, from the hood, roof, trunk, lights, and windows. Snow left in place can blow off the car and obstruct your vision or interfere with the driver behind you. In addition, a white-covered car makes it more difficult for others to see you.
- Always drive at a speed that's appropriate for the prevailing visibility, traffic, and road conditions. Failing to adjust your speed to the ever-changing road conditions is one of the major causes of accidents in winter driving. Not only snow, but sleet, freezing rain or drizzle, and dense fog can make driving hazardous and increase the likelihood of being in a multi-vehicle accident.
- If you get stuck in the snow, turn the steering wheel from side to side so that the tires push the snow out of the way. Then give the car a little gas to see if you can't begin to move slowly.

## IF YOU HAVE TO STOP

- Choose a spot where you will be somewhat protected by an underpass or the tree line. If you can't get the car to move, stay with it and wait for help.

- Protect yourself and the car by immediately doing what you can so that others will see you:

  - ◆ Set up warning triangles so the car can be seen.
  - ◆ Lift the hood; the state patrol will likely be checking for stranded vehicles.
  - ◆ Carry a red fluorescent flag (like a biker's flag) for maximum visibility.

- Use your cell phone to alert someone about your situation.
- Run the engine occasionally so that you can use the heater to warm up the car. Clear the snow from the exhaust pipe and crack open two windows for ventilation. Only run the heater for short periods of time. Experience has shown that running the heater for 10 minutes every hour is enough to keep the occupants warm and will conserve fuel while reducing the risk of carbon monoxide poisoning. If you feel nauseous or sleepy, turn the engine off.
- Leave the overhead light on when the engine is running so that you can be seen.
- Keep your circulation going by doing isometric exercises, and clapping your hands and moving your legs occasionally.
- If you're with someone else, trade brief sleeping periods. You will each need to be reawakened periodically; if your circulation slows, the risk of hypothermia increases.

According to the Colorado State Patrol, one of the biggest mistakes people make is not staying with their cars. People become disoriented and die of exposure when they probably would have been all right if they had stayed with the car. In any storm, the state police will constantly be patrolling.

## TWO TOP TIPS TO TEACH CHILDREN
## ABOUT WINTER STORMS

1. Playing in the snow is great fun, but children can still get hypothermia and frostbite. Teach them to come in when they get too cold or when their extremities start to turn pale or white.
2. Remind kids that in the storm's aftermath, they must be very careful around traffic—cars may not have good control. Children shouldn't walk in the street, and at corners they should stand well back from the street before crossing.

## HOT BUTTON

- Only go out in a storm if it's absolutely necessary, and if you do go out, tell someone where you're going and what route you're taking.
- Dress in layers and don't overexert yourself.
- Take special care when driving. Give other drivers a wide berth so that you don't slide into another person's accident.
- If you get stranded, stay with your car. Someone will find you.

# Hands-on Emergency Information:

## —Shutting Off Utilities
## —Creating a Temporary Toilet
## —To Contact for Additional Help

## Shutting Off Utilities

There are many times when turning off your utilities will be vital to protecting your life and property. If you're not familiar with how to do it in your household, the following will help, but an on-site tour and demonstration will be all the better. Ask someone to take you to your garage or basement to show you exactly where your utility connections are located, and to show you how the following information applies in your particular case. (If you live in an apartment building, see below.)

You might want to make a copy of these instructions and hang them on the wall near the electrical panel or shutoff valves.

Keep a crescent or pipe wrench in one location so that in an emergency you'll have the tool you need.

### WATER

Shutting off the water prevents flooding from broken pipes and keeps contaminated water out of the building's plumbing.

The water shutoff valve is located outdoors in areas where the climate remains warm and indoors where the climate reaches subfreezing temperatures.

Turn the valve clockwise to shut off the water.

## ELECTRICITY

When a problem develops in the electrical system, there is an immediate danger of fire or shock. All electrical systems are designed to shut off automatically with a circuit breaker or fuse. Damage to the wiring or overloading the circuit with too many appliances will cause overheating or shorted wires that should trip the circuit breakers.

To turn off breakers, flip all breakers to the "off" position.

To turn off fuse boxes, shift the lever on the side of the box to the "off" position. In the case of an old type of fuse box, pull out the cartridges in the center of the panel.

## GAS

Gas should only be shut off in an emergency. Authorities will sometimes tell you to turn it off before an evacuation. You should also shut it off if you smell gas.

If natural gas escapes into the atmosphere, there is immediate danger of fire or explosion. (Appliances that use gas may include ranges, refrigerators, water heaters, heating systems, and clothes dryers.)

If you smell gas, get everyone out of the building as fast as possible. Open windows and doors to ventilate the building and release gas buildup. Do not use matches, candles, or electrical appliances, or turn light switches on or off.

If a gas main breaks, such as under a street, leave the area immediately, and notify the fire department.

### *How to shut off the gas*

The gas valve is located on the meter, which is usually found outside on a wall, or inside in a basement or utility room.

Use a crescent or a pipe wrench to turn the valve 90 degrees or one quarter turn in either direction.

Once the danger has passed, only the gas company should turn on the gas and light the pilot lights.

## FOR APARTMENT DWELLERS

Ask about your individual apartment. Most will have separate electrical panels that you can turn off yourself; gas stoves should have a shutoff valve on the appliance itself, and some water sources (toilet and sink, generally) can be shut off from inside the apartment.

Most large apartment buildings have on-site resident staff who can respond to emergencies. In smaller or medium-sized buildings, one or two residents should be designated as emergency backup respondents (to the regular staff). They should be given keys or access to utility rooms and shown by apartment management how to turn off the utilities.

If you live in a two- to four-family dwelling, then take responsibility yourself by asking your landlord where the utility shutoffs are located, if any special tools are needed, and how one gains access in an emergency (your utility room is likely locked).

Remember, utilities should only be turned off if you suspect there is a problem.

# Creating a Temporary Toilet

If you're up against it and have no toilet facilities, here's what you will need and what to do:

● Items required for creating a makeshift toilet:

   ◆ heavy-duty garbage bags and ties
   ◆ medium-sized plastic bucket with lid
   ◆ disinfectant

- ◆ household chlorine bleach
- ◆ small shovel for digging

- ● Here's how to build a makeshift toilet according to *Talking About Disaster*, produced by the National Disaster Education Coalition:

    Line a bucket with a garbage bag and make a toilet seat out of two boards placed parallel to each other across the bucket. After each use, pour a disinfectant such as bleach (one part liquid chlorine bleach to ten parts water) into the garbage bag. This will help avoid infection and stop the spread of disease. Cover the bucket tightly when not in use. Bury garbage and human waste to avoid the spread of disease by rats and insects. Dig a pit two to three feet deep and at least 50 feet downhill or away from any well, spring, or water supply.

# Emergency Agencies

The following agencies and services provide additional information on a number of topics covered in this book. While national headquarters information is provided below, you'll find local offices or the websites to be more directly helpful.

If you need to contact the American Red Cross, the local weather service, or an emergency office in your area, check the website or your local Yellow Pages for information on the location nearest you. Each state also has a geological survey office where you can get answers regarding the positioning of your home and property.

In addition, check out the websites where you will find information on current (or pending) disasters, and in general, each makes for fascinating reading.

American Red Cross
National Headquarters
Jefferson Park
8111 Gatehouse Rd.
Falls Church, VA 22042-1203

703-206-6000

*http://www.redcross.org*

Federal Emergency Management Agency
500 C St. SW
Washington, DC 20472

202-646-2500 or 202-646-4040

The Federal Emergency Management Agency's Publication
    Warehouse, 800-480-2520
*www.fema.gov*

For a listing of U.S. state emergency offices, visit the following
    website:

*http://www.lifelink.com/statelst.htm*

NOAA/National Weather Service
Dulles International Airport
Washington, DC 20041

703-260-0107
*http://www.noaa.gov*

National Fire Protection Association
1 Batterymarch Park
Quincy, MA 02169

Has brochures and materials on fire prevention

617-770-3000
*www.nfpa.org*

For additional information on geological disasters, visit the U.S. Geological Survey website (*http://www.usgs.gov*) where you'll find information on everything from volcanoes to earthquakes. There is also a separate National Earthquake Information Center:

*http://www.earthquake.usgs.gov*

In addition, the U.S. Geological Survey has an automated fax system, Earthfax: 703-648-4888

# FURTHER READING

While this book discusses many ways to keep your family safe in various situations, you may want to read more in a few areas that are only touched upon here:

*The American Red Cross First Aid and Safety Handbook* by the American Red Cross and Kathleen A. Handal, M.D., Little, Brown.

*The Family Guide to Preventing and Treating 100 Infectious Illnesses* by Phyllis Stoffman, Wiley.

*The Gift of Fear* by Gavin deBecker, Dell.

*Protecting Your Life, Home, and Property: A Cop Shows You How* by Captain Robert L. Snow, Plenum.

# INDEX